Praise for *Mind Your Body*

———

"Nicole Sachs deeply understands the connection between trauma, the body, and chronic illness, and her transformative program can help anyone suffering from chronic pain live a better life."
—Arianna Huffington, founder & CEO, Thrive Global

"When faced with chronic symptoms, I personally applied Nicole's insights to unveil my path to healing. This book serves as a transformative road map, offering actionable steps that promise liberation and empowerment."
—Gabby Bernstein, #1 *New York Times* bestselling author

"The work I did with Nicole has been life-changing. When three separate back surgeries didn't resolve my pain, Nicole's work on nervous system regulation and her explanation of the mind-body connection opened a whole new world. I went from chronic and debilitating back pain to complete freedom, on and off the court. I can't thank her enough."
—Michael Porter Jr., Denver Nuggets

"Nicole unmasks our people-pleasing, conflict avoidance, and 'niceness,' and shows us precisely how to finally properly listen . . . and heal."
—Elise Loehnen, *New York Times* bestselling author of *On Our Best Behavior* and host of the podcast *Pulling the Thread*

"While the young mind is filled with potential, it also stores the seedlings of chronic pain. Nicole Sachs is on a mission to help us understand the brain's power to connect emotional experiences with physical responses, so that pain becomes surmountable. Her deep conviction and crystal clarity are life-changing, literally. This is a must-read not just for people managing chronic pain but also for the healthcare providers eager to help them."
—Cara Natterson, MD, bestselling author of *The Care & Keeping of You* and *This Is So Awkward*

"Filled with detailed accounts of how stressful events shape the pain we experience in our bodies and anxiety in our emotional landscapes, we learn how strengthening mental skills of attention, awareness, and self-compassion can transform our suffering, as we shift from merely surviving to thriving in a new life of freedom and choice."
—Daniel Siegel, MD, author of the *New York Times* bestseller *Aware*

"Nicole Sachs has been invaluable to me during my darkest days. Her loving and tireless care helped me heal from my trauma and loss of my beloved partner. The unbearable sciatica I suffered over five years ago has never come back, thanks to the tools I learned from Nicole. It is not hyperbole when I say that she gave me my life back."   —Ricki Lake, actor, talk show host, documentarian

"Nicole's work helped me to fundamentally change my life, allowing a gentle and brave light onto the wounds I'd buried. This book distills all her wisdom, with insight and passion, and provides a tool kit to set you free from chronic pain and anxiety. I hope the whole world reads it."

—Rachel Platten, Emmy Award–winning, multi-platinum recording artist

"A transformative guide for anyone seeking to understand and heal chronic pain. Sachs's groundbreaking approach, rooted in the mind-body connection, offers not just hope, but a clear path to lasting recovery. This is essential reading for anyone ready to break free from suffering and embrace true wellness."

—Dr. Scott Lyons, founder of The Embody Lab

"Sachs masterfully bridges the gap between emotional healing and physical well-being. With profound insights and clinical expertise, she integrates inner child work with her JournalSpeak practice, providing the tools to foster deep connections within ourselves and process our repressed emotions."

—Frank Anderson, MD, Harvard-trained psychiatrist and author of *To Be Loved*

MIND
YOUR
BODY

A Revolutionary Program to
Release Chronic Pain and Anxiety

Nicole J. Sachs, LCSW

Foreword by John Stracks, MD

A V E R Y

an imprint of Penguin Random House

New York

AVERY

an imprint of Penguin Random House LLC
1745 Broadway, New York, NY 10019
penguinrandomhouse.com

Most Avery books are available at special quantity discounts for bulk purchase for sales promotions, premiums, fund raising, and educational needs. Special books or book excerpts also can be created to fit specific needs. For details, write SpecialMarkets@penguinrandomhouse.com.

Hardcover ISBN 9780593716939
Ebook ISBN 9780593716946

Printed in the United States of America
1st Printing

Book design by Ashley Tucker

The authorized representative in the EU for product safety and compliance is Penguin Random House Ireland, Morrison Chambers, 32 Nassau Street, Dublin D02 YH68, Ireland, https://eu-contact.penguin.ie.

PUBLISHER'S NOTE

Neither the publisher nor the author is engaged in rendering professional advice or services to the individual reader. The ideas, procedures, and suggestions contained in this book are not intended as a substitute for consulting with your physician. All matters regarding your health require medical supervision. Neither the author nor the publisher shall be liable or responsible for any loss or damage allegedly arising from any information or suggestion in this book.

All names and identifying characteristics have been changed to protect the privacy of the individuals involved unless otherwise noted.

Mental pain is less dramatic than physical pain, but it is more common and also more hard to bear. The frequent attempt to conceal mental pain increases the burden: it is easier to say, "My tooth is aching" than to say, "My heart is broken."

—C. S. Lewis, *The Problem of Pain*

For Lisa,
who took the whisper of a life-changing message
and made it a roar

CONTENTS

FOREWORD

I distinctly remember the first day I ever talked with Nicole. She and I were both early in our careers in Mindbody medicine, and Dr. Eric Sherman, one of Dr. John Sarno's original psychotherapists, had suggested that we meet.

That day I happened to be in Denver, Colorado, at a somatic psychotherapy training, and Nicole and I had arranged to chat by phone. Once the training was over for the day, I drove to a coffee shop, hunkered down in a quiet corner, and called her with my brand-new iPhone.

Back then, the world of Mindbody medicine was a lonely one. There were only a few physicians and psychotherapists around the United States who were practicing under its paradigm, and no one was digitally connected in the ways we now all take for granted.

As a result, I remember my intense delight in discovering that Nicole and I spoke the same language. We swapped stories of our own healing journeys, compared notes of how we were working with our clients and patients, and realized that I had attended one of Dr. Sarno's patient panel discussions at NYU in New York City on which Nicole was a speaker.

Most importantly, Nicole and I discussed how to collaborate effectively so that people who were experiencing chronic pain and other symptoms could benefit from both of our perspectives and skills. We started talking that day about how to take a team approach to offer the best strategies of both medicine and psychology in order to help people heal in this Mindbody way.

In those early years, a number of my patients were able to tap into Nicole's amazing private psychotherapy practice in ways that were life-changing for them. I've worked with people who'd had chronic symptoms for decades, who now live their lives free of chronic pain because of the work they did with Nicole.

Since then, I've been honored to have a front-row seat as Nicole has expanded her offerings to go from working with one person at a time as a psychotherapist, to dozens at a time in her workshops, to hundreds at a time in her memberships, to millions at a time with her outstanding podcast and now this wonderful book you're about to read.

Having been able to watch Nicole's work up close over the last fifteen years, I'm so excited that you're about to experience her expertise and passion. I know that she's dedicated her life (or the nonparenting part of it) not only to spreading the word about this method of healing chronic symptoms but also to being the best of the best in helping people heal those symptoms.

Mind Your Body is an outstanding assemblage of Nicole's life's work. She makes it so easy to hear her voice and wisdom on every page as she opens you to the essential aspects of Mindbody healing and explains how to get better by employing JournalSpeak. Her energy resonates through these pages as clearly as it did that very first day we spoke—in her repeated reminders to breathe and be kind to yourself as well as in her generous offers to borrow her certainty about your healing if your own isn't yet strong enough.

As you know, chronic pain can feel uniquely isolating, as I learned many years ago in my own pain recovery and then experienced early in my career. Having Nicole as a colleague over these decades has made the field much less lonely for me, but more importantly, having Nicole as a resource has made this passage through illness much less lonely for hundreds of my patients and millions of people around the world.

I'm so excited that you chose Nicole to help guide you along your way, and I wish you all the best on your continued journey toward healing.

—John Stracks, MD

AUTHOR'S NOTE

It Needs to Be Said (Right Now and by Me)

Around the globe, hundreds of millions of people are needlessly suffering.

We come from all socioeconomic groups, genders, religions, ethnicities, and communities. The thread that binds us is that we have been diagnosed with some manner of chronic symptom or other seemingly incurable medical condition that limits us in countless ways. Often debilitated, we live a shadow life, isolated by our pain. We might have difficulty finding success at work or in our relationships as a result of this struggle—and are much more likely to experience depression, suicidality, or a substance abuse disorder. Often we have tried a variety of different drugs, surgeries, alternative and holistic procedures, and other medical interventions hoping to find even a hint of relief. Just as often, that relief doesn't come.

It doesn't have to be this way.

I've often heard the cautionary expression tossed about when people are trying to decide whether to express something challenging, controversial, or potentially misunderstood: *Does it need to be said? Does it need to be said right now? Does it need to be said by me?*

In this moment, I know the answer is decidedly *yes to all*.

If you are struggling with chronic pain or anxiety, please know that there is another way forward. I am going to teach you to be well. It's not just that I want to, I *need* to. It is imperative. The determination to do so whispers to me in the night. It pops into my mind while I'm running. It bosses me when I'm scattered and motivates me when I'm weary. Why? Because this work has created my entire life. It began by completely eliminating my chronic pain and symptoms of any kind, but that was only the very beginning. It has rebuilt my relationships. It has found and reimagined the roots of my perfectionism and codependency. It has located and healed my inner child. And, most importantly, it has allowed me to teach with the kind of presence and certainty that offers others enduring healing and personal agency. I am on my knees in reverence to the power of the tools you will learn in these pages. I am stunned daily by its stories of lives transformed. I am embarrassingly passionate in my sharing of it. I find myself, at times, despairing that I can't wave a magic wand and transplant this knowledge into the brain of every person I know.

Carrying this message has not been an easy task. There are so many nuances that can be misunderstood or resisted. Regardless of the challenge, I persevere. I have no choice. There is a greater hand at work here. You might describe it as a spiritual path, or simply say that it would be impossible to sit on such transformative knowledge without spending a lifetime sharing it.

Either way, this is fabulous news for you, because starting at this very moment, we are in it together. Stick with me and you will be astonished at what your life can become. There is no leader or guide like the one who has walked through her own fire and then circles back to take your hand and walk you through your own. My name is Nicole Sachs, and this is what we are about to do.

For the purposes of our time together, let's get some shared vocabulary down so we don't have to waste energy parsing different ways to express certain key topics. To that end, when I say *pain*, please allow this term to hold space for any chronic symptom you are experiencing, even as it moves and morphs. This includes muscular or nerve pain (back, neck, shoulder, hip, elbow, knee, sciatica, fibromyalgia, headaches/migraines, and so on) as well as any stomach issues (irritable bowel syndrome [IBS], inflammatory bowel disease [IBD], small intestinal bacterial overgrowth [SIBO], leaky gut, bloating), flaring autoimmune symptoms, tinnitus, chronic anxiety, panic, obsessive-compulsive disorder (OCD), dysthymia, and more. If you don't see yourself in this list, don't worry. They are just examples. In my twenty-five-year career, I have witnessed transformations from such a wide variety and complexity of symptomology that it would be impossible to inventory in its entirety.

You will learn in these discussions that most chronic conditions originate from a dysregulated nervous system. It confusedly informs the brain to send signals of pain, inflammation, muscle constriction and spasm, neuralgia, and other physical and experiential manifestations to "protect and distract" you from your overflowing repressed emotional reservoir. You will understand that we, often unconsciously and for years, have lived in long-term, sustained fight or flight. Our health is failing as a result. We will discuss all of this in exquisite detail, so don't worry if it is initially hard to understand or believe. I'll get you there. In the meantime, just know that I am dedicated to handing you back your life, and I will do everything in my power to do so.

We will be examining brain science, too. For the purposes of this book, I will be using the terms *brain, nervous system*, and *amygdala* somewhat interchangeably. I will also be referring to the phrase *fight or flight* to hold space for the entire fight/flight/freeze/fawn phenomenon. This is not to be reductive, nor to suggest that the complexity of these structures or processes is unimportant. Every word in this effort has been chosen with one, and only one, end in mind: *to explain in the most digestible way the intricate and remarkable activity transpiring in your mind and body.* This book is an operating manual to change your life, so let's make it easy to follow. Trust me, it will be far less bitter a pill than the many ineffective ones you've taken in the past.

We are a team now—you and me. We are joined by thousands of like-minded souls who are boldly and bravely walking this path alongside us. Each chapter will end with one of their stories. As much as possible, I have kept these accounts in their own words. I want you to hear their voices. I want you to feel their energy, their despair, their awakenings, and their gratitude. This is real life in full color—theirs, and soon yours. I want you to realize that you are no longer alone in this struggle, and you don't have to be afraid anymore.

To begin this journey, all I need from you is willingness, openness, and the intention of replacing your fear with curiosity. We will take it from there, together. I send you love, I send you confidence (borrow mine until you can cultivate your own), and I send you resolve. This may not be easy, but I know you can do it.

Yours,
Nicole

PART I

BEHIND THE SCENES IN YOUR BRAIN

LEARN AND BELIEVE: OPENING THE DOOR TO HEALING

MINDBODY MEDICINE EXPLAINED

I finally stopped avoiding fires long enough to let myself burn, and what I learned was that I am like that burning bush: The fire of pain won't consume me. I can burn and burn and live. I can live on fire. I am fireproof.

—Glennon Doyle

My trip into the fire began young. At nineteen years old, I lay on the orthopedic surgeon's table in mind-numbing pain and fear. The X-ray glowed on the screen while my mother wrung her hands beside me. We were awaiting a second opinion to explain my symptoms. My parents had taken me home from college a week before final exams when excruciating lower back pain prevented me from even walking to the bathroom, much less finishing my semester.

"I'm in agreement," the doctor said. "The diagnosis is spondylolisthesis, a degenerative condition of the lower spine. To avoid being in a wheelchair by forty, you will need to immediately stop several activities and accept certain realities. We will have to reevaluate what exercise looks like, and you certainly won't be rollerblading."

Rollerblading was a daily form of transportation that was integral to my joy and mental wellness. It was the nineties, after all. At that moment, his words directly called into question my entire sense of identity as strong, fit, and free to do as I pleased.

He went on. "It's ill-advised to lift anything over twenty pounds or ride in a car for more than an hour. You'll have to sleep in very specific positions to avoid pain and stabilize your back. Travel of any kind will need to be carefully considered from a risk/benefit analysis. Most importantly, you should come to terms with the fact that it's unlikely you will carry a biological child. The weight of the baby could strain your back to the point of irreparable harm." This last piece of news was too much to process. A life without the vibrant family I'd envisioned? Was that any life at all?

Based on what he saw on my films, the doctor explained that spinal fusion surgery was the standard protocol. But since I was young and otherwise healthy, it could wait. If I was willing to follow the strict guidelines for sleeping, travel, and exercise, I could put off the surgery as long as possible. Recovery would entail weeks of downtime and decreased mobility for life. Awash in the overwhelm of this dark prognosis, I felt that only the present seemed real. Yet what mattered most in that moment was not being addressed.

"Will the surgery eliminate my pain?" I asked in desperation. The tenor of the doctor's energy shifted as he explained that the surgery carried no guarantee of pain cessation.

For the first time in my life I realized that though they were well-versed in reading films and reporting results—and certainly wanted to help—the doctors didn't have solutions for what was most urgent: curing my pain. This was an inflection point for me. A quiet skepticism of their power to fix me, paired with the unimaginable vision of the future they were painting, became the seeds that would later grow into my desire to understand human pain more deeply. I needed to believe that there was a better way. I had no choice but to turn my attention to finding it.

Fast-forward thirty years: I am fifty-two years old, a mother of three almost-adults, and a barefoot beach runner. I travel the world, drive cross-country regularly to take my kids back and forth to college, and sleep any way I please. It turns out that this doctor, along with the many others who conferred over my diagnostic tests, was wrong. They saw an abnormality on a film and assumed, however understandably, that the finding was the cause of my pain. It was not.

First driven by desperation, then fueled by curiosity, I began a surprising and ultimately rewarding journey to discover all I could about the nature, cause, and treatment of pain and chronic suffering. It started with earning my undergraduate degree in psychology, followed by a master's in clinical social work, and culminated in the practice of Mindbody medicine in association with Dr. John Sarno's office at the Rusk Center for Rehabilitation/NYU Langone Medical Center. For over twenty years, I have been guiding people once mired in seemingly endless chronic pain, conditions, illness, and anxiety to total freedom through my private practice, podcast, retreats, and online offerings.

PAIN SEEN THROUGH A NEW LENS

For those who might not be familiar with Dr. Sarno, he was a pioneer in Mindbody medicine, a paradigm that questions long-held assumptions of the medical establishment. Simply defined, Mindbody medicine recognizes the influence that our stored trauma and repressed emotions have on the brain science behind bodily health. When an individual is experiencing a physical illness—particularly a chronic one—the Mindbody approach looks at the issue through a wider lens, seeking to understand how our physical, mental, and emotional systems are working together to keep us safe and alive.

Dr. Sarno's model challenged the traditional Western view that pain or discomfort is *directly correlated with the affected part of the body* and should be treated as such. His remarkable scientific work uncovered that real physical symptoms, including chronic pain and anxiety, gastrointestinal issues, autoimmune flares, and even dermatological problems, were not always tied to pathology or structural abnormalities in the body. Rather, unprocessed trauma, psychosocial stressors, and repressed emotions, over time, could build up and trigger the brain to send signals of illness or the sensation of injury. He referred to this condition as tension myoneural syndrome (TMS)—and discussed its impact in his groundbreaking 1984 book, *Mind over Back Pain: A Radically New Approach to the Diagnosis and Treatment of Back Pain.*

Sarno defined TMS as the process that is activated when acute symptoms like tension headaches or strained muscles morph into a chronic condition or diagnosis. In the Mindbody community, you will often hear people refer to themselves as "TMSers" or exclaim, "My TMS is acting up today!" The acronym is an umbrella term under which myriad chronic conditions reside. It includes muscular pain/spasm/inflammation of all kinds, chronic anxiety, long COVID, panic disorders, IBS, sciatica, psoriasis, pelvic pain, fibromyalgia, migraines, skin disorders, the symptoms of autoimmune disease, and many, many more. This is far from an exhaustive list—which is why, as I mentioned in the Author's Note, I will often simply refer to *chronic pain* or *chronic conditions* in our discussions. As you'll learn, it doesn't necessarily matter what specific symptoms you may be battling. The key is to understand that just as we look to the body when trying to explain why you are experiencing these sensations, we must also look to the brain science behind them.

Dr. Sarno posited a much broader explanation of the genesis of pain and other chronic symptoms. Instead of a direct link between the aching body part and a related physical origin or abnormality, he suggested that a person's psychological processes and underlying nervous system dysregulation were the catalysts for chronic conditions. When seeking a reason for pain, inflammation, immune system suppression, or any of the other many manifestations of human illness and discomfort, he explained that we need to look beyond the afflicted part of the body to the origin of the pain: the brain's attempt to protect us from difficult emotions and stored trauma.

People often laugh when I tell them that I found Dr. Sarno thanks to Rosie O'Donnell. But after my mother watched an episode of *The Rosie Show* where Dr. Sarno helped one of her producers, Janette Barber, overcome leg and ankle pain so severe that she had to use a motorized wheelchair, she told me to check him out. After reading *Healing Back Pain*, I was astonished when my own back pain began to abate.

I later became Dr. Sarno's patient, open and willing to think in new and innovative ways, and grew into a student of his work, evolving his theories and practices into ones that delivered me from chronic pain to the life I live today. Over time, I also became his colleague as he referred patients into my psychotherapy practice. It was my honor to be regularly chosen to lecture beside him at NYU, and at the end of his life, our conversations turned entirely to extending his work to a growing global audience. Dr. Sarno was keenly aware that the combination of my background in psychotherapy and my personal success story in the face of a grim diagnosis brought a powerful voice to his work—one I know he was heartened would outlive him.

THE PAIN IS NOT IN YOUR HEAD

I've often found that clients initially misunderstand the concepts behind Mindbody medicine. The primary reason is that when people are suffering, they can misinterpret its message to mean *The pain is in your head.* This understandably can make ailing people quite resistant, as they've endured physical, often excruciating, pain and chronic symptoms that limit their lives. Additionally, because of its necessary emphasis on emotional experience, people erroneously infer that Mindbody medicine is suggesting that they are mentally unstable, making up their symptoms, or somehow to blame for them.

This is not the case.

Adding insult to injury is the negative association around the term *psychosomatic*, used throughout years of literature to describe how emotional and mental pain are channeled into the body. Despite the fact that scientific studies have proved, time and time again, that our stress and emotional experiences can influence our experience of pain, the term has come to be confused with hypochondria, which, once again, wrongly calls into question the real pain and suffering of the patient. Today, most scientists avoid the term. Instead, they refer to psychophysiological symptoms—or physical symptoms that are the result of psychological processes.

Knowing how prevalent this confusion is, I want to emphasize from the start that *the pain is not in your head, but the solution is not in altering your physical body.* As I will explain throughout our time together, the genesis of most chronic conditions can be explained when you understand the way a fight-or-flight-motivated nervous system sends signals of distress to divert us from the perceived "predators" causing our suffering. You will hear me repeat this idea in many ways, as I have discovered over years of practice that this is what's required to rewire your thinking. As soon as a profound mindset shift occurs, healing is significantly accelerated.

Let's talk about fight or flight. There is no cure for the human condition, and pain of all varieties is part of it. As inconvenient as it is to be such deeply feeling beings, here we are. Intense emotional experiences are both the most joyful and most daunting realities of human life, and our health and happiness depend on being aware of their power. When we don't know how to feel our "unacceptable" emotional reactions to life (shame, despair, rage, grief, and terror), we are diverted from these challenging feelings by something that our nervous systems deem safer: physical pain and anxiety. This diversion process launches us into the brain's default mode when we are faced with danger: the fight-or-flight response.

You've likely heard of this phenomenon. The primitive parts of your brain have one vital task: keeping you alive. When you encounter a dangerous situation, the amygdala, a small almond-shaped region nestled deep in the brain, is there to help you respond in a way that will increase the likelihood of survival. It signals your adrenal glands, part of the endocrine system, to start churning out adrenaline, cortisol, and other hormones. These chemicals raise both your respiratory and heart rates, ensuring that your now-tensed muscles have the energy they need to make their next move. You might get only one chance to save your own skin, so you have to be ready!

Depending on the situation, you may run from the danger—flee. If there's nowhere to go, you can stand ready for battle—fight. But while we often talk about fight or flight as if there are only two options with the power to save us, there are two other states you might inhabit when faced with perceived danger. You can freeze and hope the predator doesn't notice you blending into the woodwork. Or you can fawn—say or do whatever comes to mind to appease the threat. Moving forward, I'll refer to this response as simply fight or flight for brevity's sake—but it's important to keep in mind that the amygdala can help ready the body for a few different responses to tension or peril.

Whether your amygdala directs you to fight, flee, freeze, or fawn, this well-documented physiological reaction is meant to last for only a short time—just long enough to get you out of danger. But when the predator you face is the repressed emotional energy inside you, you can end up stuck in this state for the long term. This is what causes chronic symptoms—because your pain or infirmity is seen as "protection" from further damage.

Think of it this way: If you broke your ankle and kept running, you might damage your bones and ligaments to the point where you'd never walk again. A broken bone causes pain as protection, so you can slow down and take the steps to heal. The same is true for myriad chronic conditions—since your brain and nervous system interpret your rising dark and traumatic emotions as a threat to your life, they will slow you down to give you time to attend to yourself and escape. A blinding migraine slows you down pretty damn quick. So does an IBS attack or excruciating knee pain. But when you train your system to safely and systematically allow these presumably threatening emotions to rise, this ancient protective response is disabled. Consequently, the corresponding chronic issues abate. It's the most astonishing and exhilarating experience. This is how I have guided people to full-body health for over twenty years, and what we will do here together.

YOU ALREADY BELIEVE

In my lectures and presentations, I have been surprised to discover how few people realize that they already connect the experience of acute pain to emotional triggers. For example, when I speak to rooms of hundreds of people, I often pose the question: "Who's ever gotten a headache after a long, stressful day?" Inevitably, every hand shoots up.

Next, I pose, "Who's run to the hospital for a CT scan of your brain, panicked it was a brain tumor?" Crickets.

"You see," I explain to the group, "you already understand that we experience physical reactions to emotional stimuli. You believe it to be true."

Although most people are willing to raise their hands and acknowledge a tension headache after a shitty day, a stomachache after the delivery of bad news, or a hive outbreak in a moment of panic, the connection between an emotional stimulus (stress) and a physical response (the symptom) is quickly dismissed when anything becomes chronic.

Chronic pain and illness are an epidemic born of fear and meaning. There is constant confusion about the natural defensive function enacted when the nervous system senses danger, and the brain responds by directing the body to protect itself. It makes sense that people are perplexed by this. After all, the "protection" is coming in the form of pain, a decidedly unsafe posture to most people. When properly understood, however, Mindbody medicine's explanation of this process brings clarity. If the nervous system deems stressful emotional experiences as dangerous predators, of course you are safer home sick! People are often the primary trigger for difficult feelings, and people are everywhere.

THE EMOTIONAL RESERVOIR

The key to dealing with chronic symptoms resides in understanding that a person's stress, repressed emotions, unresolved trauma, and smaller daily frustrations are causing *nervous system dysregulation.* As you are learning, this dysregulation is capable of inciting a range of symptoms that run from the most dramatic and acute syndromes to a simple fatigue for life. You can envision these suppressed emotions as being stored in an invisible container (picture a glass laboratory beaker), residing in the space between your belly button and chest. In my practice we call this the *emotional reservoir.* Each day as we trudge through our lives, juggling relationships, children, career concerns, money issues, and all the triggers left over from an unseen and unheard inner child, the reservoir fills little by little. Imagine a cup of liquid being poured into this space every time your kid sasses you or your boss gives you the side-eye.

When the reservoir reaches maximum density, it threatens to spill over, letting your conscious mind know about the overwhelming, out-of-control "mess" of your life. Reflexively, the nervous system switches into fight-or-flight mode. At this point, it instructs the brain to send signals to start a migraine (or a fibro flare, back zing, shoulder "pull," pinched nerve, IBS event, etc.). Once you become totally enmeshed in the symptom, its inconvenience, the dread it elicits, and the self-care it requires, the brain has done its job. You are no longer in danger of feeling that unbearable weight of life. Believe it or not, this is where the primitive brain systems deem you "safe." The triggering feelings are once again pushed down and the reservoir is temporarily calmed, as energy is expended on activities that carry a sense of control, like researching "cures" and making doctor's appointments. This, of course, is not the recipe for a fulfilling life, but for far too long, we have not considered that there might be another way.

Repression, a known defense mechanism, is not in and of itself unhealthy. Defense mechanisms are labeled as such for a reason: They seek to *defend* you against that which feels impossible to survive. It would be impossible to function in day-to-day life if you had to feel the impact of every emotional trigger. But repression with no healthy outlet cannot be maintained. Eventually, the pain needs to be felt somewhere. I often say to people, "When a tree falls in the forest and there is no one there to hear it, it still makes a sound." By this I mean that your stored trauma and unaddressed feelings bubbling underneath the surface may be hidden from your conscious view, but even if you are not listening to them, they are resonating somewhere. They are reverberating around your body as pain and anxiety like the pinball that you pull back and release, pinging from one bodily system to the next. Our rising repressed emotions are like that falling tree: Even if we don't feel them consciously, we will experience them physically. Years of watching people completely reverse this reflexive process of "confused safety" tells me so.

Most people are stunned to realize that the nervous system could be so misguided in its effort to keep us alive, but it makes logical sense. Whereas acute back pain or an autoimmune flare can be interpreted as being "handled" by rushing to a specialist or taking a medication, daily conflict and childhood pain are perceived (consciously and unconsciously) as impossible to confront. This is why chronic issues become chronic: If you believe yourself to be in control of your health and therefore safe, your system will keep you right there.

This is why I say chronic pain and symptoms are an epidemic born of fear and meaning. You are frozen in place, unconsciously terrified to move forward and disturb the "safety" that illness has provided.

Let's keep our perspective—it's kind of essential that the most primitive parts of your brain, like the amygdala, are working hard to keep you vital. Here's the catch: Whereas early humans had only predators like venomous snakes and saber-toothed tigers to contend with, modern society is a veritable onslaught of hazards. Today, they come in the form of our partners, parents, bosses, life stressors, and kids (who also, often, feel like our bosses). This is where the Mindbody dance that I'm describing enters the picture. The pain takes the place of the stressor, and you feel "in control" of your days, however miserable. Additionally, chronic states of ill health lead you to prioritize self-care behaviors that track logically with safety, like stopping to rest and asking others for support. You slow down, draw boundaries, and soften your demands on yourself.

Human beings are inherently social animals with a need for community, yet modern existence draws us away from this notion with its emphasis on independence, "powering on," and "being a warrior." Paradoxically, chronic illness and the connection it requires bring us back to an evolutionarily safe place.

So how do we stop this cycle and take back our health and our vitality? The answer lies in rewiring the nervous system's misguided reflex to protect us with pain and syndromes. Honed over years of clinical sessions and virtual work with people all over the world, my signature tool of JournalSpeak, paired with guided mindset management and self-affirming meditation, has consistently yielded staggering results. It may feel too simple to be true that exercises like targeted journaling and meditation could cause such remarkable shifts in physical health (it certainly did to me!), but it is unquestionably true. I hear dramatic stories daily from people formerly on total disability who are now back to work full time. Those who previously needed wheelchairs are running and hiking. Countless others with lesser hurdles are embracing fuller lives without consistently having to accommodate chronic anything. It's an amazing feeling of freedom. Keep in mind, it may be simple, but it's not easy. This is your work, and it will test you in ways that may surprise you. We will cover it all. Trust that the destination will be worth the journey.

JournalSpeak, as you'll come to understand, is a vehicle for healing in the form of unbridled self-expression and inner inquiry. It is a focused and specific journaling practice that teaches you how to unearth your obscured emotions by speaking from the voice of your inner child with total permission and guidance. It is the bridge between repression and a message of total safety to the nervous system.

14

I created JournalSpeak out of necessity at my lowest moment. My pain had reached the point where just mentally labeling my triggers and reactions was no longer doing the trick. I needed to go further—to find a way to solidify the communication between my unconscious and conscious minds to prevent my emotional reservoir from spilling over. The process of JournalSpeak has allowed me to access unexpected hidden places—places where my own ugly thoughts and feelings were trees falling in a forest that I had previously been unable to hear. It has also allowed me to have a part in changing the lives of others, something that never fails to move me as I hear from so many of you with staggering stories of recovery.

As you will soon see, when the impolite, unthinkable truths are exhumed and safely felt, the nervous system no longer reacts by flying into protective mode and sending pain signals. The reservoir lowers, and you shift from fight or flight to rest and repair. The chronic pain, issues, anxiety, and conditions resolve, often completely. I will explain to you precisely how to unlock the cages within which these unresolved feelings sit. This allows you to walk toward joy and presence on your own power. Each of us holds the key.

"I'VE TRIED IT ALL"

Most people who've come to me as a psychotherapist have usually exhausted all other medical and holistic paths. They've seen primary care physicians, specialists, surgeons, functional medicine doctors, nutritionists, acupuncturists, and alternative practitioners of all kinds. They've ruled out diseases or conditions like a cancerous tumor, anemia, or an untreated infection. Some of them (like the young me) know that they have options for surgery, but (also like the young me) their doctors are offering no guarantee of pain cessation. They have yet to understand what I am sharing here:

Many tests, scans, probes, MRIs, films, gut microbiome analyses, and other attempts at diagnosis reveal findings that, although logically connected, do not account for the physical discomfort and pain they appear to cause. They are "normal abnormalities," as Dr. Sarno put it, and are as likely to cause distress as they are to go unnoticed for a lifetime.

I know this sounds odd. A normal abnormality? Yet as no two bodies are the same, we all have the odd anatomical quirk. And just because a test or scan shows something *different* doesn't mean it's pathological. Take bulging discs, a degenerative condition where the intervertebral disc begins to protrude from the spine. Just the name sounds painful—and like something that would "surely" be the cause of agonizing back pain. But when researchers at the Mayo Clinic reviewed computer tomography (CT) and magnetic resonance imaging (MRI) of more than three thousand people without back pain, they found that a significant number showed disc bulges in their scans—and the prevalence of those findings increased as people got older. A whopping thirty percent of people in their twenties showed bulging discs in their films, and that number skyrocketed to eighty-four percent for those in their eighties. Yet none of them experienced back pain. So if as you read this, you think, *But my test or scan showed an abnormality!* I caution you to remember that it may not be the cause of your pain. It wasn't the cause of mine.

To be clear, I don't propose that one can melt away a tumor using Mindbody techniques. Medical interventions are not anathema to me, nor do I ever advise against ruling out something that could require immediate attention. I am a believer in Western medicine, take my children to doctors and specialists when needed, and gratefully give them antibiotics when they have an infection. In the most heartfelt way, my biggest issue with the medical model is in the despair it has engendered in the countless people with whom I've worked and interacted. Far too many diagnoses and conditions are communicated as "incurable" to those who have them. Hearing "Sorry, there is nothing we can do for you. You're just going to have to live with it" is a devastating experience, and it is far too common. Perhaps this is your experience, too.

Sometimes worse, many people with chronic pain are offered an endless cycle of strategies, supplements, new meds, and "cutting-edge" procedures that cost thousands of dollars and leave them no better for the investment. This can lead to depression and hopelessness, and understandably so. I'm not saying there's no place for these potential innovations, but using them without doing the work to get to the root cause of suffering keeps people indefinitely trapped in the pain cycle. It's like Whac-A-Mole with painful symptoms popping up in different places, demanding your attention. Maybe this is you as well.

Here's the thing: When you've exhausted the gamut of medical tests and procedures, there comes a point when you must surrender. Human beings require *a lot* of trial and error before we reach true readiness for change, and, more often than not, it's when you are on your proverbial knees that you find a path forward. The road to different is uncomfortable (you'll hear me say this once or twice). The energy of surrender and acceptance, delivered to the nervous system, is like salve to a wound. It helps you understand that uncomfortable does not equal unsafe. As you learn how to take back your power, you shorten the length of suffering.

YOUR NEW LIFE BEGINS NOW

Once the central theories of Mindbody medicine are understood, you can more readily embrace its potent healing potential. You don't need to be on your knees to heal; you just need to trust that there is a solution and use the tools to reach it. This book will serve as a road map, personal guide, cheerleader, and proof of possibility until your own physical health becomes your evidence. I will provide you with the same tools and counsel that have led to the cessation of my own chronic pain and that of so many others. I will demonstrate the power of these techniques through diverse human stories, illustrating how Mindbody practices can help alleviate what were once enduring symptoms. I will instruct you on how to do this work, and inspire you to keep going until you find your way to relief. I will call out the most common roadblocks that may foster resistance or slow the progress of recovery. And I will clearly outline best practices for your success: belief in the theories, consistency in the daily work, and an essential emphasis on patience and self-compassion.

Dr. Sarno and his theories of Mindbody medicine have thrown open a door that has changed the trajectory of my life. This paradigm has given me my freedom, my joy, and my three beautiful children. As a psychotherapist, teacher, podcaster, and speaker, I've worked to educate and inspire people around the world. And now I'm overjoyed to be here with you. This book is not about your mother, your long-suffering neighbor, or your dramatic best friend. It's about all of us. No one is immune to the pain of the human condition, *but there is a cure for chronic pain because chronic pain is an epidemic of fear and meaning.* We are all the product of systems that operate in the darkness of our unconscious (and thank God—would you want to be in charge of circulating your blood?). Being aware of how they work and using Mindbody tools to neutralize perceived threats will empower you, making you self-aware and in charge of your own destiny.

Best of all, what begins as a quest to eliminate chronic symptoms will quickly reveal itself as a path to more fulfilling relationships, heightened self-worth, and a completely new lens on life. Pain is strong stimulation and gives us vital information, yet it is not inherently negative. Although daunting and distracting, pain is the biggest littlest part. It is an invitation to recognize the truths and traumas that have been awaiting your acknowledgment. This shift in perspective will come, and when it does, it will propel you into wellness and freedom unlike anything you've experienced before.

Lieke's Recovery from Long COVID—Age 35 (The Netherlands)

I want to start with the happy ending: I am a travel journalist, a wannabe surfer, a mountain climber, and an adventurer by heart. I have my life back—living it to the fullest, surfing every wave that comes my way, and moving about the world from destination to destination without fear of illness or panic.

I tested positive for COVID at the very beginning of the pandemic. There were no experts yet, and health care in the Netherlands was only available to people who were hospitalized. Because of my age at the time and because I was able to breathe, I had to heal at home. I was visited twice in eight weeks by a doctor in a "space suit" for checkups.

Soon after the initial COVID infection cleared, I began experiencing new and troubling symptoms. It started with extreme nausea and stomach upset. After about two days, my respiratory system started to burn. My heart started racing, and I experienced severe chest pain, brain fog, and shortness of breath. I was extremely dizzy.

The weakness and dizziness made it impossible to shower. For weeks, alone, I washed up with a washcloth in my bed. I couldn't even walk from my couch to the kitchen without feeling like I would faint. I couldn't wear a bra because of the tightness in my chest and shortness of breath. All I did was lie on the couch or in bed with my arms above my head, so I could breathe more easily. This was my life for months.

I had broken up with my boyfriend two months before the pandemic, so I was alone. The news was filled with horrible statistics. There were no more hospital beds left in Italy, people were outside on gurneys in the streets across Europe, and young people were dying, too. I was at home on my own, isolated, for two months. Back then we were not allowed to leave the house with any symptoms at all.

The pain in my chest and the racing of my heart made it almost impossible to sleep. My body was unable to relax or lapse into a state of rest. I couldn't concentrate on a puzzle longer than five minutes, answer text messages, or talk to someone on the phone. The symptoms would only get worse when I tried. My every thought was consumed by my health, and I spent my hours terrified I would have a sudden heart attack.

My existence had gone from traveling the world, going to the gym four times a week, and laughing and talking into the night with friends from all over the globe to being locked inside my home for weeks in a body that didn't feel like mine. All I was left with were my thoughts, my fear, and the feeling that I was being misunderstood by everyone. Why was I sick for this long?

One evening in the midst of great despair, I had an epiphany that came seemingly out of nowhere: I might not be able to control my body, but I could take good care of my mental state. I had always meditated and valued the emotional aspects of health as highly as the physical. I shouldn't stop now! I began trying to make my home my safe space. I lit candles, meditated, practiced easy yin yoga when I could to stretch the muscles in my chest. I started keeping a gratitude journal. I really, really tried. But still, I wasn't healing. The symptoms continued to terrify me, tearing down any progress I made in my spiritual work.

Finally, eight months after my COVID diagnosis, I talked to a well-informed medic. She told me that my body was in a sustained fight-or-flight posture, and that had to heal over time. I appreciated the information, but heal *how*? Even the most well-intentioned experts were offering no solutions.

I began attempting slow walks outside around my neighborhood, at a snail's pace. One morning, I clicked on a Dutch podcast episode that featured an influencer who struggled with chronic back pain for a long time. She mentioned Nicole Sachs's podcast, *The Cure for Chronic Pain*, and how it helped her understand her body in ways she never did before. And then she mentioned her disturbed nervous system. Could my symptoms be coming from the same place?

Desperate for answers, I started listening to Nicole's podcast with an open mind and an open heart. There were no episodes about long COVID at the time (little did I know that I would be the first!), but I was struggling with unexplainable chronic pain, and that's what Nicole and her incredible guests were discussing week after week. One of the first things that resonated with me was when I heard Nicole say, "The pain is not in your head, but the solution is not in your body." She explained very clearly that when a nervous system goes into a sustained fight-or-flight posture, every perception of overload is a trigger. Mental and physical activities would initiate the symptoms. I recalled the medic who told me that my nervous system was in that sustained fight-or-flight posture.

For the first time in months, I felt like somebody was explaining to me how I could heal my body. I had always believed in the mind-body connection, but I had no idea how profound it could be. I realized I could not change my body's reactions by simply having the intention to calm my physical triggers—I had to go deeper and convince the triggers not to fire in the first place. If I could somehow teach my nervous system that emotions like fear, shame, anger, and sadness were no threat to my life, maybe the symptoms would start to soften. Borrowing Nicole's belief and the tiny fire of hope she lit in my heart, I started my healing journey.

To clarify: Long COVID symptoms are very real, debilitating, and painful. The pain is not in your head or caused by panic attacks. What I learned is that Nicole's methods help you reprogram the automatic response your body experiences when you feel these "dangerous" feelings of fear, shame, anger, and sadness. I understood that, slowly but surely, I could accomplish this and heal.

I began to JournalSpeak. Although I had journaled for years, this was a new approach. I might not be able to release my thoughts and fears solely through meditation, but I could actually sit down with them and give them a voice. It sounded so simple, but in understanding the brain science, I knew it was revelatory. As I wrote, I would listen to my fears, my anger, my sadness, my shame, and my fear of the future. In my JournalSpeak, I allowed myself to really inhabit this dread. I went to my darkest places, cried a lot, and confronted all the shadowy stuff I had been pushing down for so long. I was locked in survival mode and didn't even know it.

I sat with my long COVID experience. For months I had been terrified of dying, petrified of the consequences for my family, angry with all the friends who left me when I was at my lowest, ashamed I was not healing like most young people, and scared I was taking up too much space. I lost friends who simply did not want to talk about COVID because of their own fears. My life had changed drastically. I let myself mourn.

I also had to look at my upbringing. As much as I love my family, the dynamics of growing up were, at times, very intense. My father struggled with two heavy burnouts that resulted in a lot of tension in the house, and my brother has autism. It was nobody's fault, but at a very early age I learned how to adapt to situations and never be "too much." My feelings always came second, and I thought this kept me safe. I began to understand that when you unintentionally learn that other people's emotions are more important than your own, you become disconnected from what you are feeling. While journaling in brutal honesty, without shaming myself into having empathy for others over myself, I connected to my five-year-old self and her insecurities, fears, shame, and anger. Most of all, I acknowledged her incredible sense of responsibility for everyone else's happiness. I witnessed her constant search for safety.

JournalSpeak helped me explain (to myself!) the things I hadn't been able to acknowledge or feel before, as I'd spent all of my formative years feeling like I had to be strong, take care of myself, be positive, and protect my family. I was shocked to discover how much my mental health had taken a hit. I started practicing radical acceptance and embracing my darkness, instead of pushing it down. It was damn hard, but slowly my energy began to lift. I was able to go on longer walks. I started talking to friends on the phone. These might seem like little things, but they were big things to me.

I wrote down each win so I wouldn't forget about my progress, because healing is definitely not a straight line. Initially, every time the symptoms flared, it would push me back into my familiar, "safe" bed, and I felt like I was failing. I worried I was not doing it right, not doing enough. But I persisted. I realized that progress is dictated by the nervous system's perception of safety, and resisting my current state of being was not helping me. Like Nicole often says, "Left foot, right foot, breathe." I took her advice and befriended the fear. I gave it a seat at the table and in my journal.

My advice to you, straight from the heart: Release the need to control your pain, and try instead to observe it with love and patience. Looking back, you will see that you are not still in the same place as where you started, even when you backslide. Remember, everyone does. It's part of the process. This is our brains rewiring and learning new ways to function, and it takes time and safety.

There is no timeline for anyone's specific healing, but within a couple of months I was able to ride my bike on the bumpy canals in my hometown of Amsterdam. The symptoms were still there, but I became able to observe without fear. I was kind to myself when I needed a break. Neither pushing through at any cost nor letting fear guide me, I struck a balance. I always asked myself, "What is this pain trying to tell me? Where am I feeling conflicted? What is scaring me?" I still ask myself these anytime I feel an uncomfortable sensation in my body.

Doing this work opened my eyes to my constant fear of the future and my intense sense of responsibility to not be a burden to anyone around me. The thing is, I was panicking about all of this *without it actually happening.* My biggest challenge is to stay present. If it's not happening right now, it's not happening.

I know that recovery goes hand in hand with frustration, losing your patience, feeling like you're failing, and wanting to skip to the hallelujah phase. Just stick with it. Chronic pain may isolate you and make you feel misunderstood by many, but JournalSpeak will allow you to connect with your heart. To soften. You will slowly teach your scared nervous system that you are safe when you feel big feelings, conflicted feelings. Hope paves the road to transformation. As you do this for yourself, please hold tight to my story and all the healing stories you will hear and read. Believe that you are able to heal, too. Take up all the space you need, so you can feel safe again in your own body. You have no idea how well you can be.

Last week I was in Norway, writing about the most stunning fjords. Last month I ran on the exquisite beaches of Mauritius. All those months back, I thought I was dying. But I didn't know that I was yet to actually live. My illness, my lowest moments, and the miracle of this work have changed my life forever. Whatever you're experiencing, please know that it can shift. It has for me, and I am forever grateful.

CHAPTER 2

A WHOLE CHAPTER ON THE BRAIN SCIENCE

I was scrolling through social media the other morning when I saw that I'd been tagged in a stranger's Instagram story. When I clicked on it, I found a young Spanish woman named Matilde talking about her experience with devastating headaches. She explained that they had been going on for weeks, and when she finally managed to see a neurologist, the doctor told her that she had developed a migraine disorder as a result, he thought, of a virus she had contracted months earlier. The MD explained to Matilde that there was "no cure for migraines," but she might find relief with "very strong pills." She was frightened by the idea of an incurable condition requiring powerful medication—and the potential that she might need to rely on such drugs indefinitely. She resisted filling the prescription for weeks. Finally, Matilde relented, unable to tolerate the banging in her head.

But when Matilde got to the pharmacy, the pills were out of stock.

Returning home in a panic, she typed "chronic pain" into the search bar of her podcast app. *The Cure for Chronic Pain* appeared. She listened to several episodes, and the first spark of optimism she'd felt in almost a month was ignited. She was skeptical at first—

but with her mind opened thanks to her desperation, Matilde decided to attempt her first JournalSpeak. "Why not, right?" she recounted to her followers. "I had nothing to lose!"

On the day I was tagged in her story, Matilde could barely contain herself. After weeks of pain, she gleefully reported that this was the fourth morning in a row she hadn't woken up with a migraine. After suffering daily, she was astounded. Of course I was thrilled to be witnessing her progress in real time, but then I heard the dreaded statement come out of her mouth: *"It's so crazy that this terrible pain has been in my head all this time!"*

To be clear, this lovely girl was not complaining. Indeed, she was overjoyed. It was the first time in a long while that she had found relief and, of course, hope. But Matilde was brand new to this process, and her understanding of TMS was in its nascent stages. She had fallen into the most common misunderstanding regarding Mindbody work. Not yet educated on the true genesis of her pain and why her symptoms were relieved by the practice of JournalSpeak, Matilde figured that if emotional excavation could resolve her symptoms, then the pain must have been imaginary in some way—a construct of her mind. This confusion is so often the case. Matilde, in putting words to what so many have thought and misinterpreted, reminded me how important it is to reiterate—right up front and over and over—the pillars of neuroscience behind chronic pain. Trust me, your brain will appreciate the exercise.

Let's say it again.

THE PAIN IS NOT IN YOUR HEAD

The pain is not in your head. You are not making it up. You are not hysterical. You are not creating it. This is not your fault. You are not dramatic or overreacting. You are suffering in the same way you would be suffering if your limb was severed with a knife. Yet it makes sense that people might come to this erroneous conclusion once they've experienced symptom relief from this work. An emotional exercise that cures a physical condition? *Doesn't that imply that it was in my head?* It is essential for you that we debunk this misleading notion decisively.

Since your nervous system needs to be in the space of safety to regulate and allow the body to properly heal, taking the time and care to integrate the brain science behind chronic conditions is a worthwhile effort. You will often hear me mention that my work has three facets: *Believe, Do the Work, and Patience and Kindness for Yourself.* Like the legs of a stool, all three are required to build the kind of foundation that supports robust wellness. As you embark on the journey to address your chronic pain, walk mindfully through this important content. Doing so will create new neural pathways of understanding, helping to cement your confidence in this process and why it works. Belief is your safe passage—the door through which all healing resides. Why? Because your perception is your reality. Believing in the science of TMS sends a message of safety to the nervous system, and that is where the modern miracles of Mindbody medicine reveal themselves.

THE PAIN BRAIN

You are in pain, and the sensation of pain is the sensation of pain. The reason anyone suffers in any and every capacity is that pain signals are being fired by the brain and nervous system, landing in different bodily systems and muscle groups. To understand why these signals are working overtime in this manner, we need to ask ourselves a critical question: *Why?* Why are they being initiated?

This is where the amygdala comes in. As we discussed in Chapter One, this small, almond-shaped area of your brain is part of the limbic system, the neural network that is responsible for emotional processing. The amygdala is one of the most primitive brain structures. It has existed in human beings (not to mention all mammals) since the beginning. It may be a tiny structure, but it is mighty. This is the spot where the fight-or-flight response, our automatic physiological reaction to stressful or frightening stimuli, originates.

What does that have to do with your pain? When you break a bone, tear a muscle, or cut or burn your skin, the nerves from that area of the body send an SOS signal to the brain letting it know that you are in trouble. The brain then sends a pain signal in response. It does so for good reason. I repeat: *Pain's number one objective is to protect you.* Remember that in ancient times, when we injured ourselves in a way that required assistance, our survival hinged on getting help before we became so vulnerable that we could be attacked or eaten. Pain is the messenger, alerting you that it's time to attend to your body to avert a disastrous end.

The amygdala, which is sometimes referred to as the "reptilian brain" because evolutionary biologists believe such regions dominate the behavior of reptiles and other more primitive animals, is exactly the same as it was in our earliest relatives. Although human beings have developed far more complex and sophisticated brain structures that allow us to reason and create in constantly evolving ways, this survival hub remains unchanged. The reason the fight-or-flight response hasn't evolved over generations is that in many ways it hasn't needed to. Human beings require a lot of help getting through life, down to basic survival. Thanks to the amygdala, you automatically pull your hand off a burning pot handle before your skin melts off. In a split second, you jump out of the way before a speeding vehicle makes impact. These reactions are not something you have conscious control over—and you shouldn't! If human beings had to consider whether to recoil from something that had the power to end us, most of us wouldn't be here to tell the tale. We gratefully sigh with relief when our "catlike" reflexes keep us from injury, never comprehending that the same automatic and life-saving process is also responsible for keeping us chronically ill.

The reason for this confused protection lies in understanding the concept of *predators*. Life is full of them. Back in the day it might have been a larger animal or the flames of a fire that moved too close. Today, perhaps it's the neighbor's snarling dog or the backyard grill you realize someone forgot to turn off as you're attempting to clean it. A predator, for the purposes of this discussion, is anything that you could consciously or unconsciously perceive as a threat to your life or safety.

Back in the day, a saber-toothed tiger would be a pretty straightforward threat. If you sensed this predator approaching in the grass, you might first become very still, assessing whether it had seen you (freeze). If it began to run toward you, the brain would send messages to your adrenal glands to start pumping adrenaline and cortisol, allowing you to hopefully run to safety (flight). If you found yourself in the unfortunate situation of having nowhere left to flee, you might pick up a weapon and begin swinging it at the creature (fight). During this acute and immediate experience, your whole body would be on board to help you survive. Systems like circulation and respiration would optimize for the battle, whereas digestion and elimination would essentially grind to a halt—there is no time to worry about hunger or using the bathroom when you're fighting for your life! And obviously, although it can't be a win every time, this hardwired reflexive process has allowed humankind to continue surviving, thriving, and propagating the species for millennia.

Fun fact: If you injured yourself while running from the tiger, you would not feel any pain until you were out of imminent danger. The brain not only has the capacity to create physical pain; it also has the power to inhibit it. The nervous system will not let anything get in the way of your protection. Once that saber-toothed tiger was well out of sight, the pain would begin at the site of the injury, letting you know that you needed to attend to it. Take note again that the brain can both generate pain in the body and terminate it. It's essential to understand the different things that this incredible organ can do, especially as we examine what happens to your body when the predators chasing you aren't as obvious.

Your nervous system acts as your body's sentinel. It is taking in information from the outside world—and surveying the landscape to keep you safe. When it encounters an injury, illness, or stressful situation, it sends a red alert to the brain. You need to act to stay safe—and you need to act now! These signals may result in the brain prepping your body to fly, fight, freeze, or fawn. But it may also respond to the sentinel's warning by sending out pain signals so your body can go into rest-and-repair mode.

These processes are essential to your survival. It's all too easy to see how they work when you are faced with a hungry tiger or out-of-control flames. What's harder to understand is that the same dynamic can be triggered by the predators within us.

THE PREDATORS WITHIN

If the only predators threatening our lives were aggressive animals and searing heat, life would be a lot less complicated. This is not the case. Recall the reservoir of emotions we discussed in Chapter One. In modern society, "danger" is everywhere. The brain's evolution has allowed us to analyze, deconstruct, pre-grieve, overthink, catastrophize, or "awfulize" just about everything. As you're learning, this has created an entirely new world of predators in the form of our partners, children, colleagues, and friends, not to mention the snarling perils of money, self-consciousness, purpose, and success.

We find ourselves in unconscious conflict: *I love you, but I resent you. I want you, but you trigger me. I need you, but my childhood trauma makes that feel unsafe.* These deep, conflicting emotions build up, reach critical mass, and eventually refuse to be kept at bay any longer. As your emotional reservoir begins to overflow, these feelings knock on the door of consciousness, threatening to inform you of exactly how angry, sad, trapped, or ashamed you feel.

Your brain perceives your repressed emotional world and stored trauma as predators. It sees them *[your emotions]* as far more dangerous problems than the physical manifestation of your pain or symptoms. This is because your emotional world and the trauma you have experienced (both capital *T* and little *t*) are complex and difficult to "solve for" in the computer that is the human mind. So our brains do what we need them to do—assimilate all of the pain (other and self-inflicted) that we have experienced and pack it away for later. You will hear me refer to this often as "safe in the unsafest way." Although we have a momentary respite from catastrophizing over one issue or another, the unconscious mind can only take so much. The feelings begin rising into consciousness, sending the red alarm spinning. The switch flips, and your nervous system goes into fight-or-flight mode.

This causes the brain to search feverishly for a place to protect you. There is no cave where you can hide to keep these predators at bay. Running away won't help, either. Modern protection requires more—and illness, however unwanted consciously, is protective. It requires stillness. Illness means slowing down, asking for help, softening your insidious criticism of yourself. Illness means drawing boundaries, saying no, and staying home.

As I said, safe in the unsafest way.

Our innate wiring also convinces us that this brand of "safety" comes with an element of control. When we are micromanaging our lives to work around/fix the pain, we are back in the driver's seat. We have agency and power. We cancel plans because we're too uncomfortable to join the group. We tearfully lament the limits of our lives to the people we love, gaining empathy and connection. Although we can't possibly know this in the moment, our nervous systems have calmed down amid this unfortunate existence. And while this state may give the illusion of stasis to our nervous systems, it is a far cry from freedom.

The most effective protective posture for each person is something that you will *believe*—migraines because your mother and grandmother had them, knee pain at the site of an old injury, back spasms that concur with some (as Dr. Sarno coined) "normal abnormality" like a bulging disc or spondylolisthesis (like me!). Or, perhaps, the symptom might be related to an anxious connection that your brain has taken in—fibromyalgia described in detail in a terrifying exposé, pelvic pain that keeps your best friend in bed, anxiety and panic disorders that run in your family, or long COVID that has occupied the darkest corners of your mind since it was revealed in the press. It is equally possible that there is no medical finding associated with the site of your pain. You will learn during our time together that where your symptoms present themselves, in the end, is immaterial. As long as they grab your attention and distract you from the overflowing reservoir, they've done their job.

We know this pain is not, as Matilde confusedly expressed, "in your head." Even outside the world of Mindbody medicine, leading researchers are coming to understand that chronic pain is not merely the result of an injury or abnormality at a physical site. Many are now advocating a *biopsychosocial* model—arguing that the development of chronic pain is a "multidimensional, dynamic integration among physiological, psychological, and social factors that reciprocally influence one another."

What does this mean in plain English? Although the physical injury may have initially started with knee pain to remind you to rest while it healed, psychological, social, and emotional variables can help it transform into a chronic issue. Let's say you strained your lower back while awkwardly moving something heavy. The initial pain might rightfully be attributed to a pulled muscle or strained ligament. But no injury occurs in a vacuum. The psychological impact of any anxiety you may have about how you'll manage work and the kids while you are laid up can amplify the pain signals your brain is sending to the lower back. The social influence of your partner being passive-aggressively frustrated about having to do more at home while you rest also increases the volume. Whereas a strain would hurt for a few days and then abate, this confluence of factors can cause the brain to send the pain signals long after the agreed-upon healing time is complete.

And then, critically, there are other psychological processes at play: the deep, hidden feelings in your emotional reservoir that haven't been acknowledged or addressed. The shame left over from elementary school, where other kids bullied you for being different. Memories of your parents accusing you of faking it when you told them about the pain you were experiencing in your teen years. The rageful thoughts you (might not know you) have about being the only one who does anything around your house and how your family takes you utterly for granted.

These feelings matter—and they matter a lot. And as scientists are learning, such feelings play a pivotal role in why you experience chronic pain. I will be exhaustively redundant when it comes to this point. There is no way to solidify your belief and begin your transformation in earnest if this is misunderstood. What you are experiencing is not *in your head*. But what is happening in your head is strongly influencing your experience of pain.

As you're learning, the brain sends pain signals for a reason. It was designed to work in this way. It's important that I communicate this clearly, as there is nothing easy or light about this kind of pain. Chronic pain conditions have been labeled, studied, and treated for years. They have brought inconceivable suffering to millions. They have caused people to take their own lives. TMS symptoms are in no way "fake" or dramatically created. They are real and experienced physically. The signals/neural pathways activated to create these sensations have remarkable neurological overlap with those activated if you jam your finger or break a bone.

Everything we've discussed in these first two chapters is happening, and happening to you. I know this is true because you are a human being, and no human being is spared. Mercifully, because of their incredible influence on chronic conditions, these thoughts and feelings are not only an albatross. In the most stunning fashion, they open the door to great healing, providing an avenue to alleviate your pain and opening you to emotional wellness you never knew was possible.

FINALLY, A SOLUTION

One of the most frustrating things to me is that our society is rife with people espousing the challenges that befall us, but so rarely are we offered concrete methods with which to recover. Indeed, this toolkit is what I am holding as I stand on your doorstep.

We can shift our internal unconscious narratives. Since symptoms of all kinds are generated when the brain perceives your internal predators (repressed emotions, internal criticism, unprocessed trauma, etc.) as constant threats to your safety, they are eliminated when this misperception is corrected. Your children, although annoying, driving you crazy and stealing your sanity and any memory of your dignity, are not predators. Your shaky self-worth, fear of failure, worry for the future, and resentment of your mother for untold reasons are not going to *actually* kill you.

We just need to inform your conscious brain of this.

34

Recall that the fight-or-flight response was designed to be leveraged for very short time periods—long enough to allow us soft and chewy humans to either find safety or fight for our lives. But long-term occupation of this state is unsustainable. It's becoming clear at this point that the brain perceives safety when it lands on something it can "control." Although decidedly not the preferable *conscious* state of being, safety is the only imperative, and the reflexive and largely unconscious workings of the brain and nervous system are unconcerned with your physical discomfort. So it makes sense that physical sensations (in the form of pain and other syndromes and conditions) are sent to the body in an attempt to protect it from what is perceived as the greater "threat."

Purely physical treatments, such as drugs or surgery, may offer temporary relief, but they do not resolve the condition. This is because it is literally coming from a misguided brain. As you will see when we delve into the concept of the symptom imperative, often once one symptom is seemingly resolved thanks to some sort of medical, alternative, or surgical intervention (and the potential placebo effect, which is widely acknowledged as real among scientists), another symptom will pop up in its place if your emotional reservoir continues to overflow.

The solution, then, is to find a way to lower the reservoir. If the predator is represented by the overwhelm of neglected emotions and trauma-related triggers, the predator is eliminated when these things no longer feel so overwhelming. They say that sunlight is the best disinfectant. Here, we will go into your darkest rooms together and turn on the light. The predators of your internal world are not real snarling lions, they are only *perceived* threats—shadows on the wall. When you know how to safely and mindfully reveal "yourself to yourself" with belief and patience and kindness, the pain signals stop firing.

This is not a new idea. You may have heard of Dr. Bessel van der Kolk's best-selling book *The Body Keeps the Score*, which explores the bodily effects of trauma, particularly in soldiers who return from war with post-traumatic stress disorder (PTSD). Van der Kolk shows how these unprocessed traumas can lead to debilitating physical pain, addiction, or other chronic medical issues. If traumatic events are not dealt with, they will take a toll on your physical being.

Dr. Gabor Maté's book *When the Body Says No* comes to a similar conclusion. Maté looks at the links between stress, trauma, and addiction and delves into the connections between mental health and physical illness. And, like van der Kolk and me, he is working to highlight these underappreciated causes of physical pain. As we spend time here together, we will take these ideas a step further and live in the solution to eliminate chronic pain caused by emotional and psychological distress.

These important books likewise call out the physical expression of emotional pain and past traumas, but with a key difference. While the body is surely tallying the points and showing us the scoreboard, I believe that this record keeping is but a temporary state of being. The brain is plastic and capable of change until our last breath. No matter the trauma you have endured, it need not live forever in your body.

Most of us have been raised in the Western medical model, nearly paralyzed by the belief that physical issues require physical solutions. Although there is nothing inherently wrong with this in some situations, we must debunk this programming if we want to thrive. Although an enduring pain is felt and experienced physically, we now understand that in the case of chronic issues, rarely will altering the part of the body that is hurting be the solution. It's simply not where the pain is coming from.

If this challenges your exhausted mind, remember what we discussed in Chapter One regarding the many talks I've given to audiences from every walk of life: Most of us accept that panic begets hives, stress begets headaches, and anxiety and fear beget stomach issues like appetite fluctuation and lower gastrointestinal (GI) tract reactions. These are all emotional stimuli that elicit physical reactions. Keep reminding yourself that I am telling you something you already believe! To leave chronic conditions behind, you need only apply this same logic to whatever is ailing you and then do the work to reverse it. As I often say, borrow my certainty if you need to as you cultivate your own. I am as confident as they come.

Obviously, as I always discuss at the outset, it is essential that you first consult a doctor to ensure that medically treatable diagnoses are not the root cause of your pain, like cancer, heart disease, anemia, or infection. Yet once your bill of health is either clear or marked by a diagnosis that is deemed "uncurable," it is highly likely that nervous system dysregulation is the cause, and the methods outlined in these pages can reverse it. Many traditionally held medical tropes (e.g., bulging discs cause back pain, bacterial overgrowth causes stomach issues, food choices contribute to pelvic inflammation) are regularly challenged in my work as people, like myself, with formerly grim or confusing test results find their issues completely resolved without physical manipulation of any kind. This is possible for you, and as you stay with me throughout the course of this book, you will come to believe it.

THE SCIENCE IS ON OUR SIDE

Let's say you're still skeptical. Maybe some straight-up science will help. Pain remission through Mindbody practices and other remarkable recoveries is being documented more and more in current scientific literature. Dr. Sarno would be overjoyed. Recently, Michael Donnino, MD, a professor at Harvard Medical School, did a randomized controlled trial comparing treatments for chronic back pain. Donnino and his colleagues recruited adults living with chronic back pain for the past three months where the pain occurred at least three days a week. The study participants were then assigned to one of three groups. The first group continued their existing treatment regimens for the pain. The second group was enrolled in an eight-week mindfulness stress reduction program, where they learned about mindfulness techniques to address pain. The final group participated in a twelve-week psychophysiological intervention based on Dr. Sarno's work, where participants learned about the psychophysiological model of pain—and then explored their emotional history using Mindbody techniques.

When Dr. Donnino measured the participants' pain levels at the end of the trial, he discovered that those who participated in the psychophysiological intervention reported significantly less back pain than those in the other groups. And measures looking at how much their pain bothered them in their daily lives, as well as how much anxiety their pain caused them, dropped dramatically, too. Twenty-six weeks after the trial, more than half of the people who did the Mindbody training—a whopping 63.6 percent—reported being entirely pain-free. That led Donnino to conclude that psychophysiologic symptom relief therapy, which is what Mindbody medicine is all about, is "a highly beneficial treatment for patients with nonspecific back pain."

The power of the Mindbody approach doesn't just help with classic chronic pain. Donnino did a similar study on patients with long COVID. Not all people with long COVID experience chronic pain, but most report fatigue, difficulty breathing, brain fog, and sleep issues (all TMS equivalents). Many experience depressive or anxiety symptoms, too. Once again, when Donnino compared Dr. Sarno's Mindbody work to other treatments, he found that psychophysiological treatment helped relieve symptoms. The results led him to say that long COVID symptoms are most likely a "psychophysiological phenomenon as opposed to lingering physical impacts from the virus."

Researchers at Weill Cornell Medical Center, Dartmouth University, and the University of Colorado College of Medicine have also run randomized clinical trials where patients' chronic pain was put into remission by psychological reprocessing therapies. Another group of researchers successfully used emotional awareness and expression training to reduce symptom severity in patients diagnosed with IBS. Regardless of diagnosis, when patients were given opportunities to reprocess their repressed emotions and those powerful predators within them, they were able to recalibrate their nervous systems—and stop those pain signals from constantly firing.

If you need more hard and fast science to calm your loving and skeptical brain, I feel you. I've compiled a list of scientific studies in the "Further Reading" addendum in the back of this book. Feel free to spend as much time with these papers as you need. We have only one goal in mind: convincing your nervous system that you are safe enough to live a vibrant life without chronic illness to protect you from its vicissitudes.

The research is finally catching up with something I've known and lived for years—when people address what's hidden in their emotional reservoirs and do the work to regulate their nervous systems, their chronic symptoms abate. It's not always easy to address these buried feelings—it's actually quite challenging. But those familiar with my work know that I often say, "Life is a choice between what hurts and what hurts worse." This concept of duality may sound negative on its face, but in truth it provides great relief. Life is not "good or bad," "happy or sad," but a constant weighing of the least unpleasant option. The brain's natural protective mechanisms are no exception. We can live in pain, or feel the feelings associated with our stored trauma and repressed emotional world. Given the proper knowledge and tools, we have the power to choose.

Matilde chose. She started her JournalSpeak practice and saw her headaches begin to disappear. She may not have fully understood *why* she found relief, but by unearthing her repressed emotions, she began down the road of self-discovery, awakening, wellness, and freedom.

You have the power to choose, too. Armed with an understanding of the brain science and fueled by openness and willingness, you embolden yourself. You can learn the tools to help address your chronic symptoms and break the pain cycle. In doing so, you will join the many thousands who live free from chronic pain or discomfort. When you're ready, you can reclaim your life.

•

Gigi's Recovery from POTS, Interstitial Cystitis, and Chronic Fatigue—Age 27 (Bermuda)

My story with chronic pain and illness started at age thirteen when I was diagnosed with Ehlers-Danlos syndrome (EDS). This initial finding was not based on any symptoms per se but rather the doctor's opinion that because I was tall and underweight, it would be wise to undergo genetic testing to make sure I didn't have a more serious connective tissue disorder. Although the tests came back reassuringly clear, I began to develop the first of my chronic symptoms, which came in the form of postural orthostatic tachycardia syndrome (POTS). This involved dizziness, blood pressure crashes, heart racing, sensory overwhelm, and neuropathy. It felt, oddly, like my feet and legs were always tingling, there was a sensation of an egg cracking on my head, and I experienced crushing chronic fatigue.

My parents took me to multiple doctors across all specialties. I had every test you can think of—blood panels, MRIs, CT scans, and X-rays. Invariably, when the results returned clear, the specialists would utter the same rehearsed line: "It's just your EDS . . . it's something you're going to have to learn how to live with."

Disillusioned and searching for further answers, we expanded the search, meeting with functional medical doctors who suggested various causes, such as mold toxicity and adrenal fatigue. With every failed treatment approach, my fear increased. And, of course, my parents supplemented my panic with their own.

I was born, however challenged by my health, with an extremely ambitious personality. As I grew, I continued to get on with my life as best I could. I excelled at school, gaining a place at Oxford University and graduating with a degree in biological sciences followed by a master's of science, where I achieved the best university exam results. Although often on the surface there was no outward indication of any problems, my life was increasingly in shambles. Every examination, paper, or social outing would result in an explosion of symptoms, sometimes lasting for months on end. It was incredibly difficult for my family and friends to understand how someone who didn't look superficially ailing (and whose tests were revealing nothing) could be suffering so much.

Several months after my mum (my greatest support system) had her own health emergency, I began to develop my first set of bladder issues, arriving in the form of a slower urine stream than usual and an increase in frequency. These were soon followed by the development of severe pain. I went to the doctor with the full expectation of walking away with a diagnosis of a urinary tract infection (UTI) and a prescription for antibiotics. Culture results revealed no infection.

I was informed that there was nothing to be done. I insisted on further investigations. I spun out, desperate to control the situation and find solutions. Urine cultures were repeated, followed by specialist testing and imaging by urologists and nephrologists. With no additional findings, I ultimately walked away with a diagnosis of interstitial cystitis (IC), an incurable condition.

This diagnosis resulted in a major deterioration of my mental health. My academic research revealed that it was a condition of unknown cause, and treatment options were limited and often no better than placebo. There were even cases of people with IC having their bladders removed with no change in their symptom experience! I felt at war with my body and couldn't understand how I had pulled so many short straws in life. The diagnoses that I had genuinely tried so hard to combat had become my prison, taking away all hope of a joyous and fulfilled life.

Luckily, unlike me, Mum hadn't limited herself to reading specialized academic papers. One evening, despairing about my state and searching for something to listen to while going to sleep, she came across *The Cure for Chronic Pain*. She stayed up half the night devouring several episodes, realizing that everyone interviewed sounded incredibly similar to me. People spoke of being sensitive, naturally empathetic, extremely driven, and perfectionistic. Many with similarly severe symptoms to my own were making complete recoveries. Feeling emboldened and confident, she appeared at my bedside the following morning emphatically declaring, "I think I know what's going on! I think your symptoms are mind-body."

I almost threw my computer across the room at her, consumed by hurt and betrayal. *What did she mean, my symptoms were coming from my mind?* Did she not understand how real and physical this was? The symptoms were in my bladder, not in my head! After all my suffering she'd witnessed and endured, how could she abandon me like this? I was irate, and dismissed her out of turn.

I turned my attention instead to another major sticking point that I had recently come across—a structural hypothesis suggesting that IC could be the result of "embedded infection." Thank goodness—something that took my symptom experience seriously. I informed my mum that although I appreciated the advice, I could not accept it. Instead, I returned to the urologist and all but demanded a heroic dose of antibiotics even though my lab results still indicated that there was no discernible infection.

I took the first dose. Within several hours, my pain reduced from a fifteen out of ten to around a two. This, of course, brought me a swell of great joy and relief. Finally, an answer to my tortured search—an embedded infection. However, there was this trifling problem—viewing this miracle from an objective scientific lens, it was just a little strange. Antibiotics take twenty-four to forty-eight hours to have full effect. It's pretty much unheard of to experience such immediate results. Nevertheless, I decided that I didn't care. I had found the solution for my symptoms, and I was certainly not going to allow any silly scientific truths get in the way. I proceeded with the antibiotic regimen.

On day four, my symptoms started coming back. At first it was just a little bit, but within hours they were screaming in full effect. I was confused. How was it that I had an infection *so receptive to treatment* that it underwent the fastest reaction known to humankind, but now it was resistant to the extreme? A small voice began speaking to me from the dark corners of my consciousness—this simply wasn't possible.

In hindsight, I can say that the decision to take this final and intense course of antibiotics was the greatest one I made during my recovery. Given the trajectory of my physical response (and using my years of study and scientific understanding), I understood that my symptoms couldn't possibly be from an infection. I was out of options. I turned to Mum and surrendered to the possibility that my symptoms were the result of something related to my brain's inner workings.

I started my journey with Nicole's podcast. I listened and listened, learning about JournalSpeak and how it unearths and reveals the dark things we don't realize we're repressing. I stoked my belief with the stories of people from all over who'd healed completely. All of my staunch certainty of structural causes and concerns began to morph into equal assuredness that Mindbody medicine was the answer to my lifetime of chronic illness and pain. I didn't look back, and with renewed energy for life, I embarked on discovering what was triggering my brain and nervous system to protect me. I began to see that the symptoms were initially just the result of the underlying emotional pain, spooking the brain into firing signals of the pain itself.

Once my mindset was solidified, my JournalSpeak took off. I wrote, systematically, about my childhood, my personality that was dominated by its perfectionism and inner criticism, and the things each day that could activate me. Over time, my symptoms decreased and decreased until they were virtually gone. There is no such thing as a cessation of all human pain. Pain is the alarm bell, and sometimes we will all hear it. The question is, what are you going to do with that information?

I now know that we just need to "wear life loosely," as Nicole says. I allow my pain to come and go, change and shift, ebb and flow. It's all fine—it's just part of being alive. Doing this work has helped me reimagine my entire life. Regardless of the many diagnoses I've received over the years, I have no chronic symptoms whatsoever. I travel the world, work full time, and now teach yearly alongside Nicole and her team at the Omega Institute in upstate New York.

I always bring my mum, my adoring and adored partner in revealing and healing this complex puzzle of pain. Most importantly, I never let a day go by without acknowledging and thanking my symptoms for the wisdom they have gifted me. I am free, I am inspired, and I hope that my story will help you to challenge your own best thinking. Sometimes it's not the whole story.

CHAPTER 3

MINDSET: YOUR PERCEPTION IS YOUR REALITY

One evening, I was working from home when I heard a sudden and loud cacophony of popping sounds coming from the park down the street. I immediately tensed up, feeling my heart rate rise and my breath quicken. As the sounds continued, vacillating in intensity, I found my body preparing itself to face danger—was someone shooting a semiautomatic rifle nearby?

Some minutes later, I learned that the ruckus was the result of some kids playing with fireworks. I can't say exactly why I didn't automatically recognize the echoing pops as an innocuous children's evening activity, but in the moment my nervous system flooded my body with stress hormones to prepare me for whatever threat might be coming my way. It was protecting me, as I couldn't yet distinguish between gunfire and bottle rockets. Even after I realized the truth, my physiological systems were on high alert, and it took some time for them to return to a normal state.

I mention this story because it illustrates just how powerful your perceptions are—and how they can influence your body's responses. If you perceive yourself to be unsafe, your nervous system is going to send all the same fight-or-flight signals to your muscles and organs, even if everything is fine. I cannot stress this point enough. Far too often, we who have lived with some sort of chronic condition have been told that there is no cure for what ails us. We hear, from the very people who we hoped might provide comfort or relief, that we'll have to live with terrible pain or gut-wrenching symptoms for the rest of our lives. This naturally changes your perception not only of your body but of your abilities and experiences. It puts you in a cycle where you begin to equate symptoms with being irretrievably broken or past the point of help. Then your nervous system steps in to protect you yet again, turning up the volume and making the signals stronger. On and on it goes. And remember, it does all of this without asking for permission. Thankfully, your brain is plastic; it develops and changes throughout your lifetime. So please be consoled—no matter how long you've lived like this, you are absolutely capable of reversing it.

To fully embrace the power of Mindbody medicine, you have to change your perceptions regarding what is wrong with you and how to fix it. This may sound a bit harsh and directive, but sometimes saving your own life requires a shattering of old ideas. I know how hard this can be. We've all grown up immersed in the traditional Western medical model, and largely, by no fault of our own, we are fueled by fear. This is not all bad. A little healthy anxiety about one's physical body can be beneficial. It keeps us vigilant. We check for lumps and bumps. We pay attention to the way we feel, and catch underlying issues before anyone else could. In many ways, relinquishing power to doctors and specialists has kept us well. We rightfully trust trained professionals to guide us.

In the realm of chronic pain, conditions, symptoms, and syndromes, though, this reflexive behavior is failing. We find ourselves frustrated and stuck. We find ourselves despairing and helpless. Our perceptions (and subsequently our realities) dictate how we feel and what we think we are capable of doing. This is no way to live.

You are now at the point where you can choose between what hurts and what hurts worse. I assure you, this is genuinely a great relief. We all know that life has its painful parts, but it doesn't help to deny this or wish it to be otherwise. Every decision you make comes with some level of attendant struggle. Whether your decision is small ("Should I have that doughnut?") or slightly bigger ("Should I have that child?"), the reality remains the same: There will be discomfort. There will be struggle. There will be side effects. In each and every one of your life's choices, you are best served when you can embrace these sometimes painful features, rather than delude yourself into believing that you're a failure because you can't relish every moment.

In Buddhism the first Noble Truth is "Life is suffering." This is because humans have a great capacity for being upset about not getting what we want or about getting what we don't want. We even, sometimes unconsciously, get upset about getting what we want! It feels dangerous because everything we have exists "in time," and time erodes. It's just a basic truth of being alive.

I would love it if life could either be amazing or awful; I would choose amazing every time! This is obviously impossible. When I can grasp the reality of choice between what hurts and what hurts worse, my perceptions change. The same is true for you. You'll see that everything has some pain in it, and you'll come to accept it. Acceptance is a salve to the nervous system. This work we are doing here may be painful, but it is far less painful than the despair, hopelessness, and endlessness of living in chronic suffering. This essential question of choice touches into the purest truth: You get to choose what you think about, what you do, and what you pay attention to. You have the power to change your perceptions, and it's a critical first step in this process.

MINDSET AS FUEL

A mindset of belief in the efficacy of this work sets the stage for a shift from fight or flight to rest and repair. That's why I emphasize the brain science—it's a potent catalyst for faith in the process and it'll put you on the fast track to transformation. As we've discussed, there are three facets of my work: Believe, Do the Work, and Patience and Kindness for Yourself. As these facets are the legs of a stool, if any of them is missing, it cannot balance. As we build your stool together, we start with belief. Mindset is critical because, much like my immediate reaction to the firecrackers, your beliefs directly affect your physical experience. I perceived myself to be in danger, and my body immediately prepared as if I were. Your experience with chronic pain and conditions has altered your perception of danger, too. The human animal is the only animal that is capable of making whatever is happening "between our ears" more real than what may be right in front of us. If you truly consider yourself to be unsafe, your body will respond in the exact same fashion as if you were literally under threat.

Let's say you're walking down the street and you see a shadow lurking around the corner. Immediately, you are brought back to a terrifying movie you saw last week where the main character was jumped and beaten within an inch of his life. Given that input, it doesn't matter if the shadow is someone stopping to reply to a text message or even just an overgrown bush, your nervous system might register it as a potential threat. If it does, your brain will respond by starting this cascade of stress hormones we've discussed, which elevate your heart rate, quicken your breathing, tense your muscles, and tell all the other systems in your body to prepare for fight or flight. You are organizing to survive whatever attack is coming.

Can't you just feel it? All of this happens whether or not the shadow represents a real predator; the body responds the same. As you round the corner and finally realize that the shadow is just a tree you hadn't noticed before, your systems will begin to calm down. It may take a few minutes, but just like the flip side, the perception of safety is all that's required to defuse the fight-or-flight mechanism and allow you to regulate. This notion is why mindset is so key in this work. Your perception is your body's reality. And your chronic symptoms have changed your perceptions of your world.

I am not here to blame doctors, your concerned best friend, or your hand-wringing mother. But once the experts have told you that you're out of options, your own experience begins to tell you the same. A state of extended panic or fear (because you can't do the things you used to enjoy) makes the world feel increasingly smaller. You might feel like a disappointing parent or partner because your pain is keeping you from fully participating in your relationships. Maybe your work has suffered. These things build on one another, leading you to perceive your own existence as a threat. When you identify your body, your pain, or your symptoms as dangerous, your physiological systems are going to respond to them in that way, too. It's an endless, negative progression.

I know I am being repetitive, and it is intentional. Resetting your mindset gives you the power to override your confused nervous system. You are evolving in real time! This is incredibly formidable stuff. Let's go over the different possibilities for optimal mindset to position you best for transformation.

BELIEVE THAT THIS WORK . . . WORKS

Best case: If you can, adopt the belief that an emotional exercise is directly connected to a physical transformation in your body. From my many years of doing this, I can tell you without a hint of hesitation that it is. Feel free to borrow my certainty until you can secure your own. Remember, as you forge this path for yourself, that there are so many supports from which to draw strength. Marinate in the energy of the brain science, my personal story as it unfolds, and those of your fellow travelers in the pages of this book. Sit quietly with the ease that comes alongside not being alone. Your lovely system will learn to trust.

When we suffer, we suffer the same. The mother who stands over her dying child is the same whether she is in a state-of-the-art hospital or a refugee camp. The man who can't get off the floor, paralyzed in back pain, is the same whether he's the CEO or working in the mailroom. The teenager who is sidelined with crippling anxiety is the same whether she's the valedictorian or the wall-flower huddling in the shadows. Physical issues bring us all to our knees, and that's why everyone's story is your story as well. This is a cause for celebration. You are a member of the human race, and we can all help each other be well. Reiterating this point is one of my missions. I bring you an army of people vast and varied, living completely new lives as a result of understanding this work and doing it for themselves. You are now among them.

YOU HAVE THE POWER TO DECIDE

Keep in mind that all profound shifts in life come from making a decision. There is great power in the inflection point that occurs when we simply, without resistance, decide to do something differently. Decisiveness is emancipation. Your decision need not be based on "logic," as logic is susceptible to the preconceived notions of what has been true for you in the past or what stands as the societal norm. Here, I am proposing an act of revolution. I am the motivational speaker on the stage jumping up and down and shaking you out of the haze of your prior shackles. *Get your hands up!*

We are going to change your life! This is the energy that fuels the kind of decision-making we are discussing here. We are here to fuck shit up.

Since your nervous system is manipulated and adjusted based on your conscious input, making a decision to believe is the gatekeeper to progress. Belief is the prerequisite for putting an end to "what was" in favor of "what's next." You begin to trust by hearing other people's stories, and then that confidence is solidified by doing the work necessary to allow your body to be your proof.

If you can't bring yourself to believe at this very moment, just suspend your disbelief. When we keep doing what we're doing, we keep getting what we're getting. And whatever you've been doing has fallen short, so here we are. This is no cause for shame. For years I was circling the same problems with solutions that didn't work, so make sure to operate with patience and kindness for yourself. If you want to begin this process in earnest and need a little time before you are honestly able to connect an emotional exercise to your physical health, then let's try manipulating your brain a little bit. Let's try taking a vacation from your skepticism, like we do when we go to the movies.

When I lecture on this, I like to tell the story of my childhood experience with the movie *Field of Dreams*, starring Kevin Costner. If you haven't seen the film, it's about an Iowa farmer named Ray Kinsella who is inspired through "divine visions" to mow down his crops and build a baseball field on his land. He is facing bankruptcy as it is, and everyone thinks he's gone off the rails. Still, Ray can't resist the urge to follow his gut. He doesn't know why, but he can't shake the "knowing" that this unhinged act will lead to everything he wants and needs in life. The story culminates as the completed baseball field attracts deceased players to come back to life and play on Ray's diamond, one of which is his father, with whom he never found a connection when he was alive. Ray not only begins to heal from one of his childhood wounds but discovers a source of endless income as people from everywhere travel to Iowa to witness the games! A tad unlikely, I'll admit.

Whether you like baseball, or believe in reincarnation, is not the point.

The point is that it's a pretty crazy premise for a movie, and I think we can agree it's improbable it will happen to any of us. It was also nominated for three Academy Awards, provided excellent entertainment, and created the kind of joy and wonder that is capable of inspiring countless human feats—none of which have any relation to dead baseball players or Iowa farms. *My* point is, if you walked into that movie and crossed your arms and said, "There's no way I can possibly believe that any of this stuff could happen!" you would waste two hours of your life. To learn from or enjoy fantasy films, we suspend our disbelief. We allow ourselves, even if for only an hour or two, to be inspired and ignited into our *own possibilities*. This can't happen if you stay stuck in what you currently "know" to be true. When you suspend your disbelief, you enter the space of curiosity. You make room for an experience to touch something deep within you. You open yourself to the prospect of previously undiscovered motivational energies.

The only way to engage in new things is to either believe they will matter or decide you're willing to be curious. As we spend this time together, I invite you to set aside fear, skepticism, and the protestations that have protected you in the past. Gently release views of what you "know." We've always needed to do this to break through. Think about life before penicillin. Think about a life limited to a flat Earth. To make progress and evolve, we need to challenge our assumptions. People have been transcending the commonly held beliefs of a culture at the intersection of every revolutionary change that eventually transforms the world.

Your other option, if you are still struggling with mindset, is to borrow my belief. I have enough certainty about the results of this work—based on my own experience as well as that of many others I've witnessed—to go around.

One of my clients, Laura, was someone who had great trouble believing that Mindbody work could do what dozens of doctors had been unable to accomplish. She came to me out of desperation, riddled with several debilitating chronic concerns. She was in such fear—and in so much pain—that she was unable to accede that this work might benefit her. She was just too scared. All the prescriptions and procedures that had promised so much had done so little.

To help her move past her fear, I got out a stack of index cards. Together, we wrote the name of each of her chronic diagnoses down on a single card. I then handed the cards back to her.

"These are yours. You do not have to give them away. You can hold on to them for as long as you feel that you need to," I assured her. "But as you are ready, and as you are comfortable, you can let me hold them for you. I will keep them safe. I will make sure they don't get lost. I know that all of these symptoms come from the same place—a dysregulated nervous system—and I will cradle them gently for you. You don't have to worry; *I am not afraid of them.*"

For far too long, Laura had felt safety within her diagnoses. I know this sounds odd—but think about it: After she was diagnosed with chronic migraine, she had a clear path of what she "needed" to do. She had to fill her prescription, take the pills, and rest. She had permission to cancel her plans and close the shades. She was allowed to draw boundaries and say no to her overbearing mother. It was a similar story with her gastrointestinal issues before that. After her Crohn's diagnosis, she'd taken the meds and changed her diet. She'd reduced her food variety again and again, even when the pain persisted. In some small way these actions had made her feel safe, in control. However, Laura was bereft. This was no way to live, and she was still in daily enervating pain. To shift her path, Laura had to decide that she wasn't defined by these conditions. She needed to access the belief that she could get better, despite so many setbacks.

At first, Laura just looked at the cards. She honestly wasn't sure which ones she could hand over. These labels sheltered her; they gave her a sense of agency and identity. "That's a hard thing to let go of," I comforted her. "Take your time, look each card over, and ask yourself if you might be willing to let me take care of it for a while."

Lovely Laura was hesitant, and I know sometimes it helps to lighten things up. "Don't fret! My work comes with a one hundred percent misery-back guarantee," I told her. "You can have any of these conditions—and all of the things connected to it—back whenever you want. But to do the work and have it change you, you'll need to relinquish them for long enough to watch yourself transform."

Laura paused for a moment more, and then haltingly handed me the card that read *multiple chemical sensitivities (MCS)*. She had been diagnosed with this condition because it was believed that certain smells would trigger migraines for her. Yet when I asked her to borrow my belief, she realized that smelling cleaning products didn't *always* result in pain.

"Sometimes I smell that floor cleaner we use and it does nothing to me. Sometimes I get a whiff and have a migraine for three days," she said. "Maybe MCS isn't the reason I'm sick." *Yes.* This is the inflection point I'm talking about. This was the beginning of freedom for Laura.

Little by little over the next few months, Laura handed me all of her cards. Once in a while she would sheepishly grab one back with a half grin, and I gave it to her willingly. After all, I had told her it would take as long as it took, and I was in no rush. By the end of our time together, Laura walked out of my office symptom-free. She no longer associated herself with the myriad diagnoses she'd been assigned for years, and she was living a life that exceeded anything she'd imagined. By borrowing my belief, Laura had found her own.

You can borrow my belief, too. Like I said, I'm as certain as they come. And I am as patient with you as I was with Laura, all the while knowing that belief is the key to starting this effort in earnest. When you falter, remember that confidence in the process greatly reduces the reflex of your nervous system to launch into fight or flight. It changes your perception of your body and your symptoms. It transforms the way you respond to all the things that happen in your life.

I have been asked many times, "How is this work different from the years of therapy in which I've endeavored to work through my issues, triggers, and trauma?" And my answer is always the same: Your therapy has been essential. Your time has not been wasted. But until you consciously connect this emotional excavation to the cessation of your physical issues and crippling anxiety, your brain has no choice but to continue protecting you. Your perception is your reality (have I mentioned this before?). When you mindfully attach reducing your emotional reservoir to the end of chronic issues, the pain signals stop firing. As you do this work, you and your nervous system will learn that you are safe to feel your feelings and gently invite your traumas to have a seat at the table. All parts of you are welcome.

Now, for a moment, let's flip it around. You've had chronic back pain for years. For as long as you can remember, every time you felt the slightest twinge, you began to spin out, reacting with fear and assigning meaning in the form of dread. What if, with the help of this book and your new mindset, you were able to decide that you were safe no matter what? What if you could get curious about the science, become willing to trust the stunning success stories, and open yourself to the possibility that the Mindbody connection is at the heart of your suffering? Your nervous system would listen to that, too. Your plastic brain would evolve and start to respond with equanimity. This is empowerment. You have so much more influence than you realize over your physical and emotional health.

So let's make a decision. Regardless of the fear that tries to whisper its directives, let's say, "Nope. Not today. Not one more day. I am ready to be brave. I am ready to be different. I am ready to replace my fear with curiosity and believe—whatever that looks like for me at the moment." Your new life awaits, and I'm right here waiting to take you. Let's go.

•

Jonna's Recovery from IBS, Migraines, and Chronic Back and Neck Pain—Age 38 (Spain)

I've struggled with chronic pain almost all of my life. In early childhood I was diagnosed with irritable bowel syndrome (IBS); I had an often severely upset stomach that seemed to reject most foods. By age eleven, I started having migraines. I remember feeling overwhelmed with school and always pushing myself to achieve more and get better grades.

Although I am sure my parents did their best, I didn't feel heard at home. My complaints, of both physical and emotional distress, were met most times with the sentiment that I was oversensitive and needed to shape up and be stronger. I was validated mostly for my achievements and being a "good girl." I paired this compliment with not expressing my feelings and having few needs, I knew it was valued in my family when you were easy to deal with. Early on, I perceived that expressing big emotions was unsafe and could deprive me of love. This was especially true of my relationship with my mother, and I strived not to create distance between us. I internalized the mindset and belief that there was something inherently wrong with me, and that love and acceptance depended on being someone different, someone better.

In retrospect, I know that getting the headaches gave me a place to rest and be cared for. I remember many times when my mother was called to pick me up from the school nurse, where I had been taken to rest as the migraine was so strong. She would come for me, care for me, and give me a pill. She would let me stay in her bed, which felt wonderful. I remember the relief I felt in the midst of the pain. Even then I knew how the headache provided the opportunity I so desperately needed for attention and care.

As I transitioned into my teenage years, I struggled with an eating disorder and an obsession with exercise. Skipping a physical routine would induce anxiety and stress. Controlling my weight and working out provided the only momentary relief I could find. I felt like two distinct people. One was excelling at school, sociable, and popular. The other was locked within herself, at home, depressed, lonely, and out of control. As the years rolled on, I continued to push myself. I was a perfectionist, an ambitious person who went to business school and became a leader in all of my pursuits. I know now that my relentless pursuit of success came from a belief that being different—and achieving more—would finally lead to happiness.

At age twenty-six, I relocated abroad, where I dealt with an exhausting twelve-hour workday in a fast-paced professional environment. I navigated the best I could to live in a country where security was always a concern. During this time, I had a car accident and almost immediately fell into a terrible spiral of pain. It initially began in my back, then radiated to my neck, right arm, and eventually my right buttock. I started to experience round-the-clock pain and eventually extreme anxiety. There was a sense of desperation that was overwhelming. My life became more and more limited, and I couldn't function without strong pain medication that would only momentarily numb the agony. I distinctly remember the heart-wrenching moment when I had to ask my boyfriend to release my hand because his touch sent searing pain through my arm and neck.

I embodied the energy of "victim." I felt as if my world had been stolen from me, and I was overcome by hopelessness and anger that this was my life. I couldn't shift my mindset—I was too afraid and powerless. I went to the doctor again and again and was eventually diagnosed with a misalignment in my neck. The orthopedist theorized that it was the root cause of my widespread pain. In desperation, I underwent neck surgery followed by six months of intensive physiotherapy and rehabilitation. The pain ceased temporarily, and I was certain that the surgery had worked. That is, until I started an ambitious new company and life became stressful again. Almost on cue, the pain came back, just as bad as before.

At this point I started the journey of trying "everything"—I saw so many traditional specialists I lost count. I had another surgery (on my back), took more strong pain medication than I dare to admit, and went to countless physiotherapists, osteopaths, spinal experts, and so on to control my pain. I was told by most of them that I would probably experience pain for the rest of my life; they could offer nothing other than things to "control it." They predicted I would never lead an active life and could forget about activities like running. I had injections in my back twice a month, yet I was still in agony and barely managed to work and live a normal life.

When I discovered Nicole's podcast, the real turning point began. Worn out by all the conventional paths, I became desperate enough to search for novel ways of approaching chronic pain. As I listened to her teachings, it dawned on me that in the brief time I was pain-free I was not immersed in a stressful environment. I know now that avoiding stress is not the answer, but that spark of realization was important in waking me up to new possibilities.

I researched more about Nicole's work and Mindbody medicine. I began to see that my pain served as a protective shield, guarding me against impossible self-expectations and the turmoil of unexpressed emotions. I looked back on my upbringing, understanding with compassion that I thought it was more important to be liked and approved of than it was to be authentic. Sickness had been a sanctuary, offering me respite from the relentless stress and pressure I imposed on myself. I recognized that my migraines afforded me the love and attention I craved from my family. My neck and back pain mirrored this dynamic in adulthood.

Through six months of dedicated commitment, I experienced a remarkable transformation. It began with a mindset shift—I was *not* a victim. I was simply human, and I had been repressing my emotions my entire life. The introduction of JournalSpeak allowed me to express myself fully, without judgment or restraint. The shift was mind-blowing. A year in, I was completely free from chronic pain, medications, and treatments.

Five years later, I live a life so full that it's almost difficult to recall the days when I was in debilitating pain. This journey has not only restored my physical health but also granted me self-awareness, self-love, and genuine freedom—life beyond my wildest dreams during the darkest days of my pain. I live without limitations, engaging in activities like running a few times a week and maintaining a consistent routine of weights and cardio. I am healthier and stronger than ever before, with no physical constraints holding me back. My back and neck pain are distant memories, and there is no hint of an eating disorder or distress if on a particular day I can't get to the gym.

I'm so grateful that this experience has allowed me to become the best version of a mother and wife. During my daughter's early years, the pain prevented me from physically carrying her and hindered my ability to be a good parent in many ways. Today, I can be there for her without exception, and with a full heart and mind—a gift to us both. My family's whole life has been transformed by this journey. I even brought my husband all the way to America to attend Nicole's Omega Institute retreat last summer, an experience we both cherished.

Occasionally, when symptoms resurface, I recognize it's time to look inward. I return to JournalSpeak and grant myself respite from life's daily stressors. But that's okay! There is nothing to be afraid of. As Nicole reminds us, "Sometimes you feel things in your heart, and sometimes you feel things in your body, and they are literally interchangeable." Physical pain, like a passing headache or a back spasm, is just a different way to *feel*. I remain gentle with myself. I don't expect to be perfect anymore. I just expect to be me.

PART II

THE WORK THAT TRANSFORMS

PREPARE: LAYING THE GROUNDWORK FOR OPTIMAL SUCCESS

CHAPTER 4

SOME QUESTIONS TO CONSIDER ABOUT YOU

Like many new parents, when I had my first child, I was freaking out. I picked up nearly a dozen different parenting books, scanning each for the wisdom that would get me through. One, *Secrets of the Baby Whisperer* by Tracy Hogg, had a line that has stayed with me decades later: "Start as you mean to go on."

In terms of getting your baby to sleep, eat, and live the most comfortably during those infamous first few months, the book's idea was to start building the habits today that would benefit you and your child in perpetuity. The goal was to avoid any future "unlearning" as much as possible—to begin with the most studied, proven, and reliable methods out there. The same applies to this work. As you prepare to integrate these Mindbody practices into your life, be extremely thoughtful about where you find yourself. There is great benefit in taking stock of who you are, what you reflexively do, and how you might be instinctively tempted to sidestep discomfort. This kind of self-knowledge helps avoid common pitfalls and lays the groundwork for optimal success.

You may wonder why I'm asking you to begin here. *Why can't we get straight to JournalSpeak, healing, change—the transformation you keep promising me, Nicole?* I understand. But it's important to recognize that by taking the time to lay the groundwork, you are in a superior position to get the most out of your Mindbody work. You are preparing the soil for growth. You are making the effort now to build a strong foundation. The next three chapters are specifically positioned to help you do this—to start as you mean to go on.

The process begins by asking some crucial questions. You must become aware of the patterns and habits that are (however unintentionally) helping to keep your emotional reservoir filled to the brim. This preparation is necessary because your brain is wily. It will whisper resistance in your ear, using your own voice, and compel you to perpetuate activities that keep you stuck right where you are. This process is normal, as the brain naturally seeks familiarity. Luckily, we are in this together. I will arm you with every tool you need to combat stasis. You've been sitting in the same place long enough.

Since you picked up this book, I suspect you've grown tired of all the ineffective efforts that've left you exhausted, drained, and still hurting. Trying something new is frightening, so we offset that fear with the power of preparation. Together we can ascertain your automatic self-soothing strategies. For example, what kind of excuses do you regularly make for yourself? What behaviors (however negative) do you perpetuate that might alleviate your stress and make you feel "better" in the moment? What kind of diversions do you attempt when you're uneasy or trying to manage big feelings like worry, regret, or fear?

Some of us head straight for the pantry, searching for comfort food. Others might pour a big glass of wine. Maybe you zone out in front of the TV or scroll through social media. However innocuous, even heading out for a long run or finding reprieve within the pages of a book can be forms of avoidance. The essential inquiry here is: Where do you go when life starts to be too much? Even things that you deem healthy can be obstacles if they are automatic. Mindbody medicine helps us to understand that nervous system regulation hinges on the opposite of what might seem like self-care in the moment—we need to *stay in the discomfort* long enough to unmask it. We need to prove to our brains that we don't require pain as protection.

As you start to consider your personal patterns, don't judge them. They are not inherently disruptive, and I'm not looking to take them away from you. But it is critical that you become awake to them. Because while they may not be detrimental—in moderation, many of these activities range from enjoyable to beneficial—you may be engaging with them in an unconscious or semiconscious manner. This can slow down your healing. You have choices and, whether you are aware or not, you are constantly making them. We take the opportunity, here, to be aware. Awareness is the gateway to any measurable change.

As we engage in this gentle, curious inquiry, we should also investigate any self-assigned labels. Do you explain away certain habits by insisting you're a "morning person" or a "night owl"? Maybe you label yourself lazy or, alternatively, a person who can't sit still? Do you define yourself as "conflict avoidant" or a "fighter"? These kinds of self-descriptors are a form of armor, as they allow us to excuse ourselves from activities that may challenge those beliefs. We may unconsciously hide behind these characterizations to avoid difficult situations. Again, none of these narratives are necessarily good or bad—but it is important that you be cognizant of them.

As you begin to consider these queries, it's normal to feel defensive. This is a natural reaction, especially when you might worry that your self-soothing strategies will be regarded with judgment. Or, worse, that they mean you aren't capable of change. This is not the case. When you can examine the coping strategies and labels you've been using to protect yourself, you are empowered to find a new way forward. My experience has shown me that if nothing changes, nothing changes. If you keep doing what you're doing, you'll keep getting what you're getting. I could pile on every other annoying cliché that touches on this idea, but I think you understand. Don't make me pull out "It is what it is!"

This effort to shed light on your unconscious escapes is a powerful exercise, and one that is worth the discomfort. There is nothing more disheartening than feeling like you are, once again, spinning your wheels. As you'll hear me say a lot, I stand in constant defense of you—in response to the threat of you. Thankfully, those who care about me command the same post in my direction. There is nothing more loving, if done with compassion.

THE BRAIN SCIENCE OF HABIT

Habits and resistance are security blankets. Even if they feel absolutely terrible, we will reach for the same self-soothing strategies again and again. Even more concerning, the ones that don't feel as terrible become justifiable in our protective brains and can keep us stuck for life.

There's good reason for this—and it all goes back to brain science. Our brains really are amazing organs. They govern every thought, feeling, and action we take, every second of every day. As a result, the brain has to keep track of an overwhelming amount of information. To make this job more manageable, it appreciates a good shortcut. Neural shortcuts are designed to help us build habits: regular, settled behaviors that don't require conscious monitoring or input. By cementing specific pathways and patterns, the brain doesn't have to consciously monitor everything we do. We can move forward, almost as if we're on autopilot, and get the job done.

Some of these habits can be as simple as brushing your teeth before bedtime. Others may be more complex—like meal prepping on Sunday nights or heading to the gym straight after work. What all habits share is that, over time, they become automatic. They free up computing power in our brains so that we can concentrate on the bigger things.

Think about what it would be like if your brain had to consciously manage something like brushing your teeth. Your inner voice would have to remind you of every little thing about the act—much as it does whenever you learn something new. Walk to the bathroom. Grab your toothbrush. Put the toothpaste on the brush. Put the toothbrush in your mouth. Brush the front teeth. Brush the back teeth. Rinse your mouth. Rinse the brush. Rinse the sink.

Once you've done a habit regularly for some time—most experts say about three weeks—it begins to become second nature. You no longer have to think about the nuances of toothbrushing. You don't even have to remind yourself to do it. It is part of your bedtime routine. This allows your brain to focus on other things: how to prepare for the next day's big meeting, remembering to add toothpaste to the grocery list, or listening to your partner as they share their day with you.

Habits, of course, are not limited to grooming or feeding. You also develop habits to deal with stress, and these habits similarly become automatic behaviors. They have you reaching into the fridge, heading out for a run, or firing up your favorite social media app before you even realize you are avoiding something. They are there to lessen the load on your nervous system. When you consider your go-to self-soothing strategies, understand that they are not your fault. The brain seeks familiarity. It feels safer to do what has been done before, regardless of the real-world result. If the brain perceives an activity as "safe," it will prompt you to do it again and again rather than risk the uncertainty of something new.

Let's talk about something that most people consciously know is a waste of time: scrolling through social media. Although it's clearly without much measurable value, it serves as a way to avoid "dangerous" tasks like getting a paper done or completing a deliverable for work that might trigger feelings of self-doubt or unworthiness. Over time, it becomes something you gravitate toward reflexively. Your fingers move toward your smartphone without a mindful decision. You click your icon of choice, and you're off. Almost immediately, your brain stops worrying about the task you're trying to avoid. Every new piece of content that flashes on the screen grabs your focus anew. Even when you acknowledge, in the very moment, that scrolling like this is a dumb thing to do—it works. I cringe to admit how much I do this myself!

This is why when we are attempting to change our lives, we must be wide awake from the start. Your automatic behaviors may have kept you "safe," but they are also getting in the way of discerning the unresolved feelings that underlie your chronic symptoms. To move forward, we must examine every potential unconscious barrier and take it seriously. This may feel silly at first or like a waste of time. I promise you it is not. This exercise is integral in opening the door to what's next. Let's do it.

TAKING INVENTORY

Invite in every label, excuse, habit, diversion, addiction. Grab a piece of paper or head to your computer and list all of the things you do to avoid feelings of discomfort or lack of control. (Keep in mind that most control is only perceived. We have so little power over what happens in life short of our own actions. Most of us have some inkling of this, and this insight alone makes us even more uncomfortable and running for relief!)

Think about the things you do when life gets to be "too much" and write them down. Maybe your avoidance takes the form of procrastination. Perhaps you tend toward trying to solve other people's problems, or zoning out to TV. Food is often an easy comfort. Some manage to dodge their worries by cleaning the house or going shopping. Drinking, using, porn, WebMDing . . . be as honest as a person who's saving their own life. Whatever your "go-tos" are, just note them. Once you've created as comprehensive a list as possible, look carefully at each item. One by one, pick a behavior and put it at the top of a fresh page and say, *Hi. I see you. Do you want to talk to me about why you're here? How are you helping me? I am ready to listen.* Keep going until all of your major players have been heard.

As you let each behavior speak, you'll see that it has lots of interesting things to say. For example, one of my go-to escapes is exercise. When things become stressful, I lace up my running shoes. If I were to ask exercise what it is doing for me, I know it would start by telling me how it improves me mentally—my thinking becomes sharp and clear after a couple miles. It also makes me feel better physically and helps me feel tired enough to sleep at night.

But if I kept asking why, I know that running would reveal other purposes. It would probably acknowledge that because I can convince myself that it's "healthy," it can't possibly be bad for me no matter how I'm using it. This narrow view, however, could ironically keep me paralyzed.

Intentionally inquiring further allows for a more honest dialogue. It helps me to understand that running also aids me in avoiding the things I need to do, like getting started on projects before the last minute. It allows me to put off uncomfortable tasks, like paying bills or having a hard conversation with my kids or partner.

This curiosity does more than just help to avoid barriers to entry in doing the work—it starts to lay the groundwork for more profound healing. The motivations you uncover at this stage can open your mind to what will provide fodder for a robust Journal-Speak practice (much more on that to come). Back to my exercise habit. In the preceding description, I noted that running might keep me from "uncomfortable tasks, like paying bills." But why, exactly, does paying bills make me uncomfortable? I have the money in my bank account to pay them. A deeper dive reveals what's underneath—I grew up with financial insecurity. My father was irresponsible with money and it affected my entire childhood. Because his choices caused pain and suffering when I was younger, any financial matters make me feel anxious even if they are ostensibly "safe." This is an important insight! It has led to many essential explorations and revelations as I've traveled down the river of my own healing. It's also unmasked many repressed emotional stories and eliminated myriad TMS symptoms. Looking at where, why, and how you avoid everyday tasks can expose essential truths that will be key in your ongoing transformation.

So take some time to inventory all of the behaviors that might be keeping you from uncomfortable feelings. Be as honest as possible. *Start as you mean to go on.* After you've created this list, look at each item and ask it, "Why are you here? What are you doing to protect me? [etc.]" Write down what comes to you as you consider each one. And remember, there should be no judgment in whatever answers come. This exercise is simply about taking the time to know yourself. It is the first step in creating an appreciation of your patterns and habits so you can be more aware of the pitfalls that may be standing in the way of your growth. If your questions about a particular habit evolve into revelations, like the one about my bill-paying avoidance, go with it! This is a project to be undertaken with an energy of curiosity and wonder. You are deepening your most important relationship, the one with yourself.

STAYING CONSCIOUS

You'll often hear me say, "The life you save is your own." In this momentous process, sometimes you need to shake things up. When this feels counterintuitive, remember: The brain seeks familiarity. You've developed these habits for a reason. They protect you— even if they are contributing to you being "safe in the un-safest way."

Shaking things up is undoubtedly uncomfortable. As you probe your habits, you may touch places that scream, "But this is the way it's always been done!" and resist any further interrogation. Receive any protests gently and with self-compassion. Your brain is on your side—it is simply misguided. You are no longer a scared, helpless, unmoored child. You are a grown person with agency, and you have the ability to change anything that is no longer working for you. Continually comfort that little kid inside—we are not looking to alter anything until you are ready, but we must seek to understand.

Keep consciously reminding yourself that no one is taking anything away from you. Reiterating this fact to your brain is vital so you can accomplish this exercise with curiosity, not fear. We are just looking at things for what they are. In her book *White Hot Truth*, Danielle LaPorte suggests, "Transformation begins with the radical acceptance of what is." I wholeheartedly agree. And if transformation begins with the radical acceptance of what is, then obviously we must understand "what is" to initiate change. In my many years of living this work and practicing it with others, I have found this to be a powerful truth. We can overcome our barriers to healing by allowing each of our habitual behaviors and labels to share their excuses, to tell us why they are here. When their objectives are revealed, we can more easily partner with ourselves in this recovery effort. The shift can be remarkable.

In so many ways, human beings are all the same. We celebrate the same, we suffer the same, and we learn the same. Our incentives are ubiquitous, as are our challenges. Taking the time to unmask the barriers to healing is an enormous catalyst for your success. It will set you up for a powerful space of healing, allowing you to look—without shame—at the ways you've been living. This act will also solidify your belief in the process. It will ready you for the simple (but not easy!) work that will help you leave chronic pain behind forever.

YOU'RE IN GOOD COMPANY

For years, with people in my office, with little smiling faces in boxes in Zoom rooms, in huge venues at in-person retreats, and even in the virtual landscape with people I've never met, the results have been the same. My recipe is in-depth and at times strenuous, but it is effective. The cake at the end is just gorgeous. Translation for the moment: These methods have been tested, and they work. But they require thoughtful reflection and solemn effort. *You are challenging your brain's habituated patterns, and it will challenge you back.* But that's okay; you are evolving in real time. My personal mindset: It's a privilege that this work is mine to do. I don't have to do it; I *get* to do it. I'm not BSing you when I say that I feel lucky, even in the grossest, cringiest moments. I have the power to change my own life.

Deep breath. An inventory is simply a list of what is in stock. It's impossible to know for certain what you need to add or subtract before you know what you have. We are here to understand your patterns and habits—and to accept that the road to different is uncomfortable. Always remember that uncomfortable does not equal unsafe. At first, it might be frustrating, or even frightening, to look at ourselves in the way that this work requires, but don't get stuck there. Ultimately, this moment will empower you to find the motivation you need to heal. And the results will be worth it in ways you cannot yet imagine.

*

Suzanne's Recovery from Fibromyalgia, Neuropathy, IBS, and Chronic Lyme—Age 45 (Northwest United States)

My symptoms encompassed my whole body. It felt like every system was affected by this mystery illness that had control of me. The sheer range of diagnoses had our heads spinning for over a decade.

To start, I had very intense and violent gut symptoms, which later were categorized as IBS. They became so severe I was receiving IV nutrition and medication to keep my weight stable. Then there were the neurological symptoms—dizziness, blurred vision, muscle tremors, ringing in my ears, a metallic taste in my mouth. I felt like I had hot water running down my face. I felt like I had ants crawling on my hands and feet. I had word recall problems, which were incredibly frightening to me. I would hear myself describing certain things to doctors and think, *Gosh! This sounds like lunacy.* I had random and unexplained joint pain, and a lot of skin stuff—blisters, rashes, hives, yeast infections. I had reoccurring urinary tract infections.

The first diagnosis that I received was fibromyalgia. At the time, I had two babies, and we were broke. We'd already spent so much money chasing after answers and trying different things that, I have to admit, the diagnosis felt like a relief. I was like, "Oh, we have a direction!" Until I learned, well, that direction is nothing. Doctors had no idea what to do. They put me on an antidepressant. I was told to try to relax more, which is decent advice. But it was hard because at the time I was just so bereft, so ill, so impacted by my symptoms. My husband and I kept searching, and he was by my side through all of it. We were raising little kids at the time. It was a lot.

The symptoms continued raging and changing, and I was diagnosed with a connective tissue disease, which falls under the category of autoimmune disorders. Yet again, not really anything to do about it. By this time I had traveled to a couple different states looking for help, desperate for relief. A friend recommended that I be tested for Lyme disease. I found a specialist in Seattle, and sure enough, a positive test. I felt so much better! I finally had a diagnosis that made sense and the bloodwork to prove it.

There was a treatment, and I hit it hard. I took high-dose antibiotics, some IV and some oral. There were times I was on three or four antibiotics at once—and *so* many supplements. Anyone who's been down the road of chronic Lyme can tell you about the supplements, I mean hundreds of them. My symptoms lessened but didn't go away. I tried all kinds of strict elimination diets, to no avail. It was then that I was told I also had *neurological* Lyme, which they thought might account for my bizarre symptoms. But—boy! That can really scare you when a picture is painted of "bugs in your brain." I couldn't get the images out of my head.

In the process of all of this, we lost our house. We had tremendous medical debt. You can infer what this level of stress was like. Still, at the time, the Lyme diagnosis allowed me to feel hope for myself again. I clung to the notion that eventually, once the next course (and the next course, and the next) of antibiotics was done, I would be free of my chronic illness at last. This only lasted a few months. It fell through my hands again, like sand. The symptoms just came back with a vengeance. I may have had Lyme on paper, but treating it did nothing for my pain.

This was real despair. The intensity of symptoms I was experiencing had completely taken over our lives. We were back in the cycle of searching for answers, which was *so* deflating. For the first time, I was afraid I was dying. I described the sensations as feeling like I'd been poisoned. It felt like something terrible—an utter emergency—was happening in my body and no one could help me. It got even worse when I realized, "Oh, it's actually *not* going to kill me. I just have to live like this." I had these two kids to raise and we'd spent so much money. I had to work! It was a very panicked feeling.

I was on the treadmill of the medical model, whether it be Western medicine, natural treatments, even spiritual work—just a full-on sprint for thirteen years. The diagnoses piled on: extreme environmental sensitivity, acute food intolerance, mold toxicity, porphyria. My world got smaller and smaller. My mental health and emotional stability were at an all-time low. I was raw all the time. I didn't hate my life. I had two beautiful children and my husband, who is the most beautiful soul. But thoughts of suicide crossed my mind. They gave me a feeling of power, as everything felt so out of control and dark. We had searched so hard and for so long.

By spring, I was at my breaking point. I can't even remember how it happened, but I came upon Nicole's podcast. It was the kind of coincidence that feels like fate. I was standing in the kitchen, just barely on my feet, trying to melt cheese on English muffins to provide some sort of dinner for my children. All I wanted to do was lie back down. I started listening, and this woman's story grabbed my attention. Her symptoms did not match mine exactly, but the science behind what she was experiencing . . . my mind was blown. I texted my husband: *I'm listening to this podcast. I think I'm on to something, but I don't trust myself. I'm so desperate, I feel willing to jump onto any bandwagon. Would you listen to this for me? I need validation that I'm not crazy.*

My husband was training for a marathon. He went running the next day, headphones on, podcast downloaded. He came back in tears. It makes me emotional, even at this moment, because our lives changed that day. I had been waiting for this shift for so many years. I had been devoid of hope, but my husband was not. He wrapped me in a hug and said, "This is it. You've got to go all in."

I dove into TMS work. I had been introduced to some brain

retraining programs in the past, and I very much believe that we can rewire our brains. This concept of neuroplasticity was exciting, and it was the evidence I needed to fully buy into the process. I became able to shift my thinking—*the solution was not going to come in altering my physical body.* I was like, "Okay, the solution is in my brain." As soon as I completely aligned with this notion, I began seeing glimpses of proof.

Within the tiny bit of safety I felt in understanding TMS, even in the midst of those dark days, I picked up snowboarding. I know this sounds completely insane. But my husband had snowboarded for years, and there was one day where I was kind of on an upswing, and our kids had a rare weekend with their grandparents. He said, "I want to teach you to snowboard. Let's seize the day. We don't know about tomorrow. You feel okay in this moment, let's go."

And this was huge. I said yes. At the time I said no to a lot. But as the years had progressed and I was trying to figure out how to live with this thing, I learned to say yes when I felt like I could. I had a lot of fear, but armed with my willingness to believe in this work, we went up to the mountain.

All the while, I was doing the work. It gave me a different way to see my symptoms when they got bad. When they flared, instead of becoming terrified—*How bad is it going to get? How long am I going to suffer? Do I need to line up childcare?*—I could just say, *I know what's happening, and I know what to do about it. My nervous system will regulate when it's ready.*

Over the following weeks and months I kept going, growing stronger. I'd get on the chairlift up the mountain every chance I'd get. I would wind myself down, and I felt alive. Symptoms would still be present, but I could do it. I described it to my husband like this: "It's like the beauty and the activity distracts my brain enough that I can't fixate on the symptoms. I'm having to focus on getting myself down that mountain!"

The first few setbacks I experienced were hard. My brain could flip that switch so quickly. I went into fight or flight, and the symptoms were instantly severe. But I soothed myself. I did my Journal-Speak and meditation. My husband cheered me on. There were a couple times he just said, "Don't give up. Please, this is it. Keep going. We've already seen a difference."

And I did keep going.

Today, I consider myself recovered. After thirteen-plus years of widespread, debilitating, life-altering symptoms, and all the diagnoses, I am a healthy, active person. I teach school full time. My kids are now twelve and fifteen, and I am very involved in their lives. My husband and I both work in education, so when summers come, we are able to be very active. We make tons of travel plans—tomorrow we are going to a concert out of town. And wait for it . . . last weekend my husband and I ran a half marathon! I'd always enjoyed jogging before my symptoms took hold, and it has been a joy to bring it back into my life.

As Nicole always mentions, I'm still myself. I still deal with anxiety. I still have sensations that come up. I still "run stressful" and want things to be perfect. But when they're not, I don't obsess. I invite all the feelings onto the kindergarten carpet. It makes so much sense to me—I have that rug in my own classroom and we sit on it every day! Everyone comes in, the neuroses, the hang-ups. And I just say, "Here we are." This work has given me my life back, and trust me, I live it.

CHAPTER 5

EXPECTATION SETTING IS EVERYTHING (OR OVERCOMING RESISTANCE)

They say, "Expectation is the root of all heartache."

In my years of life and practice, I have found this to be an undeniable truth. When we get it into our heads that something is going to be easy and it's not, it's only human to fall into the deep morass of self-pity. I have swum in these waters many a time. So as we begin this process of recalibrating your nervous system to adjust the ways in which it protects you, we need to take a hard look at the journey ahead. We need to talk about what it's going to feel like.

Straight up: You are going to face some resistance. And that resistance, in many cases, will come directly from you. The call is coming from inside the house.

You may have already encountered some of it as you worked through your habits inventory in the previous chapter. After all, your nervous system has been working hard to keep you "safe in the un-safest way." As we move toward changing your patterns—or adding new ones that help you keep your emotional reservoir from overflowing—you may find yourself struggling. This is natural, and to be expected.

That said, the energy of Mindbody work should be gentle. We are not looking to create sweaty palms or clenched fists. But there are common resistance themes that emerge as you unearth old traumas and rewire the ways you respond to various triggers. As part of the groundwork, let's lay out clear expectations of both the promises *and* the pitfalls. Knowing them in advance provides an edge and can help you manage those tricky anticipations that, unchecked, might devolve into excuses not to do the work. As I won't let you forget, you're saving and creating your own life here. Let's make every effort to eliminate anything that could block your success.

Remember that your nervous system has already decided (without seeking your counsel or permission) that your repressed emotional world is a predator capable of eating you alive. I use hyperbolic language here deliberately. The stakes perceived by our most primitive systems are not light! Knowing this makes it easier to gather the strength to fight any reflexive resistance that might arise. When you are battling chronic conditions of any kind, your emotional reservoir has reached maximum density and is spilling over, flooding your mind and body with rage, shame, terror, grief, and anything else that has been long unattended. The result is a switch that flips inside you, keeping you chronically in fight or flight. Mindbody work has the power to lower the reservoir, allowing for rest and repair. The body naturally seeks healing, but this overflowing reservoir is blocking this organic process.

Let's talk about our grumpy and scared little friend, resistance. As we began unearthing in the last chapter, resistance will whisper to you in your own voice. It is cunning—and it knows exactly how to manipulate you. It will provide you with excuses to avoid the work. It might manifest as exhaustion or impatience—trying to convince you that you lack the strength or time to continue. It may come to you as symptoms, sidelining you in an attempt to warn you that you're in danger. It often embodies a compelling inner voice, parroting all the people (including the experts) who have told you that your condition is "intractable" or "incurable." What a huge pain in the back!

And. What a huge opportunity to know yourself more profoundly and invite in the badassery you will need to transform this whole thing. (Go you.)

There are many forms of resistance that you might encounter, so we take the time here to call them all to the carpet. Similar to challenging your self-soothing strategies, we do this from a place of empathy, not judgment. We take the time to dive deep because it's vital you recognize resistance for what it is: confused inner diversions that can get in the way of pursuing this lifesaving work.

RESISTANCE AS EXCUSES

Resistance to doing the work is natural. Your inner voice, which can be so convincing, will whisper all sorts of excuses. As you cultivate awareness of the voices and the tricky ways they try to get your attention, you can neutralize their power. It's time to build familiarity with this influence. Let's seek to understand it so you can treat it as you would a child who is afraid of a monster under the bed. Resistance responds best to self-compassion coupled with firm resolve. You need to believe that you are safe to do what needs to be done.

Remember: Resistance is just another form of TMS. A moment of fierce resistance is exactly the same as a sudden headache or back zing. It distracts you from the work at hand—looking at the emotional pain and struggles for which your current symptoms have been holding space. It is the nervous system trying to warn you that it's "more dangerous" to walk into your own dark rooms of repressed emotion than it is to endure something with which you may feel more familiar, like another fibro flare. This misdirected protection can keep you stuck in patterns that make it harder to tend to your emotional reservoir.

Beneath most resistance is fear. The voice inside your head starts to panic. It tells you:

This is too much.

You have been through enough—you can't handle one more thing.

If you think about these unpleasant feelings, you will feel terrible for the rest of the day.

This is not a good idea.

Nicole's work may be effective for other people, but you're different.

You're sicker. You're too far gone.

Let's see what's happening on social media (or on Netflix, or in the kitchen, or in your work email inbox) and get to this later.

We each have our own unique flavor of this voice, but its messages share a similar energy. As you think about the excuses you make to avoid stress and discomfort, you'll probably realize why I asked you to inventory your typical patterns in the last chapter. They are, in their own way, acts of resistance. The more you can live in the light, the more effective this work will be.

Resistance in the form of excuses is a powerful barrier to healing because it is fortified by shame. Human beings are shame-generating machines. It may have started with your mother, or your coach, or the mean teacher who "hated you" in third grade. But it has continued over a lifetime in the form of self-flagellation. Shame is heartless in its messaging. The voice continues to whisper:

The Voice of Shame

You are lazy.

You are a failure.

You're never going to get better if you don't do what you said you're going to do.

You may as well give up.

You never come through.

You can't prioritize—there are more important things to do with your time.

It won't work.

This is really stupid.

You just don't want to.

Your friends would think you were crazy if they knew.

You've already ruined today so just start tomorrow . . . if you're even capable.

Here we are. This inner dialogue exists in varying degrees in every one of us, me included. So instead of heeding its whispers, let's simply *expect* them. When you are armed with right-sized expectations, you become a warrior ready for any battle. Even when you feel like you don't want to do the work, that you "don't have time," or that this "can't possibly change" you, you can recognize that *those feelings are not facts.* That voice, as familiar as it may be, does not tell the whole story. Because of your overflowing emotional reservoir, your nervous system perceives you as safer in your chronic condition. Your job in these moments is to recognize resistance—and speak back in another, more awake and purposeful voice:

"Right. Yes, I hear you. This feels like a heavy lift. This feels like a drag. This feels like it won't work. But I have power, and I've made a decision. I know this has worked for so many, and I am sick and tired of being sick and tired. I don't want to live in pain and chronic anxiety, so even if this *feels* unsafe, I'm going to believe that it's actually not. It's uncomfortable. I am learning here that uncomfortable does not equal unsafe. I am committed. I am strong. I am capable. I hear your warnings, and I appreciate you for trying to help, but we're doing this now."

RESISTANCE AS EXHAUSTION

There are times when I sit down to do my JournalSpeak and I become so physically exhausted that my eyelids feel like they weigh a hundred pounds. It comes out of nowhere. Only moments before, you might have found me full of energy and ready to go. It's a story

I've heard from tons of people. As all chronic pain originates from the same place, a misguided nervous system, so too does all resistance. This form of bizarre and immediate exhaustion is just another mask it can assume. So, just as with resistance as excuses, we simply stay aware of this phenomenon.

As we discussed in Chapter Two, your nervous system acts as the body's sentinel. It is constantly on guard, ready to help you overcome any potential threat. Sometimes it responds to stressful situations with pain signals to let you know it's time to hide in a cave and rest. Alternatively, it can also simply "wear you out" to arrive at the same outcome. When the body is dealing with an injury, illness, or other issue, the brain sends signals to the adrenal glands to let loose a flood of cortisol and other stress hormones to put you into fight or flight. It elevates your heart rate, quickens your breathing, and tenses your muscles. This takes a lot out of you. That big push for survival is, literally, exhausting. When you are in a chronically stressed state, you will, more often than not, find yourself in a chronically tired one. The nervous system is just trying to get you to pause so you can build up the energy to take on the next predator.

When you begin your JournalSpeak practice, the danger signals that accompany a perceived need for protection may fire, leading to the fatigue we are discussing here. As you encounter it, you will see that the experience of "resistant exhaustion" has a different flavor than that of other scenarios. We all know the sensation of abject physical exhaustion: the morning after an all-nighter, a red-eye flight into a different time zone, the workday that follows a night of insomnia, even the chronic daily "I'm so beat" that seems to define human existence. The resistant kind of tired is different—it's attached to nothing specific and makes no logical sense. It comes on boldly and can be very insistent that an immediate time-out is imperative.

Sure, you *feel* tired, but where is this sensation coming from? That's right—your nervous system. We certainly do live in a society of the perpetually tired. And yes, of course, you are likely not getting enough sleep. But your drowsiness isn't due to a lack of rest. Pause. There is no saber-toothed tiger waiting outside the door. Just your Mindbody work. Recognize your fatigue for what it is. Because, as I have found in my years of practice as well as in my own life, seeing exhaustion as resistance to facing difficult challenges offers an essential paradox: It helps you face them. The seventeenth-century Dutch philosopher Benedict de Spinoza is famous for saying, "I can control my passions and emotions if I understand their nature." When you understand the nature of exhaustion and resistance in general, you can keep walking when these sneaky energies tell you to give up and sit down.

RESISTANCE AS SPIKES IN PAIN

As you begin to confront your internal predators, you may initially experience some worsening pain or anxiety. This does not happen to everyone, but it is certainly worth mentioning. Some people call this an *extinction burst*. Others simply sigh and say, "Sometimes it gets worse before it gets better!" This occurrence is nothing to fear. The nervous system is doing its job and enacting protection until safety is assured. Since the primitive brain sees taking to your bed with a migraine or experiencing a flare-up of chronic symptoms as "safe," this spike in unpleasant reactions can persist without the proper understanding and perspective. Or worse, it can make you give up and run back to more pills, procedures, and tests. As crazy as it sounds, this heightened or changing pain is an encouraging sign of progress. When things get worse, it's the nervous system poking you harder on the shoulder, asking, "You okay? You *sure*?"

Yes, you are fine. The inner conflict triggered by doing the work will pass, and you will gain confidence and momentum as you begin to feel the results. Your body will become your proof.

If pain flares, meet this experience with the same energy you used with resistance when it took the form of excuses or exhaustion: "I see you, I hear you, and I appreciate you. Protection is your goal, and you want to arm me with all the security I might need. But you are just a confused child, and I am a big, confident grown-up. I know that more pain means you are screaming your directives at me even louder, and I gratefully receive them. But now I'm going to forge ahead, as everything I want in life is blooming in the flowers around the next bend. On we go!"

RESISTANCE AS GIVING YOUR POWER OVER TO "EXPERTS"

The traditional model of Western medicine teaches us to disempower ourselves. When we are ill or in pain, we learn, from a very early age, that we are to hurry to doctors and specialists. They have the knowledge, and they will make us well.

Certainly, if you have a treatable condition, you should see a physician. You should see as many as necessary to feel as if you've exhausted the medical route. This is useful for your physical health, of course, but it is also imperative in quashing the doubt that resistance brings. I am adamant that everything I teach here comes *after* a full checkup to make sure you don't need something I can't give. If you've been diagnosed with a cancerous tumor, you need a surgeon and an oncologist. If you have something that falls under the TMS umbrella, a shift in your brain's behavior can only be effective once you've taken the steps to ensure that the condition doesn't require a medical intervention.

Resistance in the form of giving your power to experts, however, is when this seeking continues after all reasonable routes have been explored. It is born of the confusion that comes from interacting with the medical world while chronically ill. As most experts do not offer a cure for chronic pain, the origin of our relations with them is fraught. We grow up believing that physicians are godlike, yet far too many of us living with chronic symptoms have felt dismissed or disappointed by the very experts who were supposed to care for us. This lack of results can be terrifying and sometimes enraging. Clients of mine have reported that they didn't feel supported or guided when a particular treatment wasn't working. Or perhaps they did, but the only retort from their doctors—however kindly intended—was that they should "learn to live with it." Sometimes experts imply that you should ignore your experience or intuition in favor of their less-than-hopeful prognoses, insinuating that your inner knowing does not have value. The fear generated in these interactions can produce a significant roadblock to getting well.

Even after you begin Mindbody work, this fear can be pervasive. It whispers to you as resistance does—in your own voice—telling you to keep making appointments, seek fourth and fifth opinions, or try a new alternative treatment or diet. I've been watching people dance with this dynamic for years, making it harder on themselves. It is legitimately hard to trust that, indeed, it is *you* who has the power to heal yourself. Here's the thing: That power is available only when you stop doubting it. The sooner you halt the hamster wheel of new "cures," the sooner you will see changes take hold in your life.

Another group of well-meaning people fall into the category of "expert" and can stand in the way of your progress: your friends and family members. These troublesome spokespersons' stories can provide different insinuations or labels that may ultimately get in your way. Think about how we often try to rationalize our chronic symptoms:

Migraines run in my family.

My best friend has tried every elimination diet known to humanity to help her IBS—maybe I should try one more.

My grandmother had pelvic pain, too.

That woman from work suffered for years with unrelenting back pain—didn't that back brace help?

I should try _____ (fill in the blank with the treatment of the day that resistance offers).

These stories shape how we perceive our symptoms—and what we think is possible to do about them. They are yet another way we can inadvertently give away our power. Then there are the advertisements, the influencers, the "helpful" neighbors and acquaintances who offer their take. They, too, will tell you stories that may invite you to fear the worst-case scenario.

When you are living in a fear mindset, you are incredibly susceptible to others' beliefs. I say this with tremendous compassion and empathy. When you're stuck in pain, it's all too easy to look for answers in the wrong places. I've been there. Just remember that when you entertain the specialist's musings that your condition is incurable—or take on your grandma's struggle as your own—it is yet another form of resistance, and one that can keep you from doing the work you need to do. It's time to widen your lens and start believing what is possible. You may not have gotten the memo, but now I'm here to deliver it: The real expert is you.

RESISTANCE AS THE SYMPTOM IMPERATIVE

TMS moves around. It's one of the most extraordinary things about chronic pain that is rarely discussed in medical circles. This lack of visibility is likely because doctors and other practitioners don't make the connection between the myriad symptoms that define chronic conditions. The gastroenterologist is unlikely to assume they're treating the same condition as the orthopedist. The *symptom imperative*, a term coined by Dr. Sarno, points to the fact that it's immaterial how TMS shows up. Some people present with headaches, others with stomach issues, still others with muscle spasm, neuropathy, or inflammation. So when you experience a new symptom or say that you feel the pain moving around from the right side to the left, *this is normal and should be expected.* You are not sick or broken. It's just more proof that you are experiencing TMS, and it is not dangerous. As you do the work with belief, and patience and kindness for yourself, the TMS will shift and eventually subside.

Let's delineate this concept more so you can prepare yourself for its crafty ways. As you move forward and commence this work in earnest, you may be tempted to perceive your progress as linear: "I had back pain, I've done the work, and now it's gone." This is often the case, but nearly every person's journey will eventually be marked by a dance with the symptom imperative. Here is how it might look:

I had terrible back pain. It owned me and directed my choices and the way I lived my life. I found this work and started doing it consistently with belief and self-compassion. The back pain began to ease! It was so great and incredible. I had been nearly free of back pain for a couple weeks, and

*the craziest thing happened. I started getting daily head-
aches that really sidelined me . . .*

We interrupt this dialogue to call out the symptom imperative.
Often in this journey, once the nervous system has begun to recalibrate and the original symptom goes away, the unconscious fear
will rise (after all, it's been your bedfellow for a long while) and
send another completely "unrelated" symptom in its place. Do not
allow this to deter you or spike your resistance. It's totally normal.

The best part of the symptom imperative is that it can solidify
your belief that there is nothing structurally wrong with you. How
could you need back surgery to be well when your symptom could
be so readily replaced with migraines? In TMS circles we call this
having the pain "on the run." As much as it may feel less than optimal in the moment, please let me assure you that you are on your
way out of the woods. It doesn't matter if there is a diagnosis attached or how "hopeless" a doctor may have deemed it. TMS comes
from one place and there is only one solution: Lower your emotional reservoir to regulate the nervous system.

RESISTANCE AS WATCHING THE CLOCK

While we are talking about walking out of the woods, let me take
the opportunity to call out one last form of resistance: needing to
get better on a timeline. If it took you five years, twelve years,
twenty-two years, thirty-seven years to walk into the woods, you
are not going to walk out in a couple months. This is not to say that
you won't make major improvements, both mentally and physically. But I have found that people who watch the clock and compare their journeys to those of others struggle far more. They
unconsciously invite resistance in the form of frustration. When

you are frustrated with anything, it is because you want it to come faster and more easily. Unfortunately, this kind of frustration makes you more vulnerable to giving up altogether. So let's expose this natural pitfall here and now: This is going to take as long as it takes.

It may seem counterintuitive, but the slower you go, the faster you get there. Just breathe. You are on your way. You were born with a certain nature that contributes to every way in which you experience the world. In addition, you have faced your own unique traumas and struggles. No matter where this finds you, you are on the right path. Stay the course, and you will feel a shift.

Always remember that the most important message to send to a dysregulated nervous system is one of safety and calm as you do the work to restore order. Urgency carries the opposite message. Think about it this way: Desire to be different than you are at the moment is translated by your nervous system into the feeling of fear. When you "need" to change to be "okay," it comes with a wave of panic. This is because we are inherently aware that change is not something that can be forced.

Urgency looks like this:

I have to be done with this. It's been so long!

That other woman who seemed just as stuck as me is posting success stories now! What the hell?

I need to get past this, or I'll never be able to take that trip for work.

My symptoms have already taken so much from me. I cannot miss one more of my daughter's recitals!

Not only is this energy the perfect storm for frustration and resistance to the work, but it also adds so much more stress (rage, grief, despair, shame, terror) into the emotional reservoir. The best posture as we move toward total wellness is *acceptance* (much more on practical ways to embody this soon). Whereas urgency communicates fear, acceptance relays a message of safety.

Acceptance looks like this:

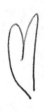

I know that this is hard right now, and I hate it. I don't want this pain and I also don't want to do the work to eliminate it. I resent the fact that the doctors couldn't help me and this job is mine. But here I am, and I am doing it. Some days it feels like I'm getting somewhere, and other days I feel totally stuck. It doesn't matter, though. I know where I'm going, and I know I'm on the right path.

Acceptance should feel like a long exhale, a release of that tight grip on your outcomes. Keep in mind that acceptance does not equal agreement. You don't have to *like* what's happening. You just need to accept it. In the world of "what hurts versus what hurts worse," I think you'll find acceptance to be the far less painful option in the long run.

YOU ARE EXACTLY WHERE YOU NEED TO BE

Human beings have what Buddhist teachers refer to as a *monkey mind*, an inner voice that swings from branch to branch trying to make sense of our experiences and find security. Ram Dass, the famed American spiritual leader, took the metaphor even further, describing it as a drunk monkey, stung by a scorpion, and then spun around until it's dizzy. You can imagine that with a mind that is inherently chaotic, it only becomes more so when you're frightened!

Pause, breathe. You are exactly where you need to be. When you know what to expect from a situation, you can anticipate your anxious mind's desire to flee from anything new or uncomfortable. When you understand that your physical conditions are the result of a misdirected attempt to protect you from "impossible feelings," you can begin to open to the alternative: *The only way out is through.*

Every day you are making progress—even when you don't feel it. Recalibrating your brain takes time. Let's say it again for your potentially beleaguered system: If it took you years to walk into the forest of your life, your habits, and your coping mechanisms, you cannot expect to walk out of it in days or even weeks. But you will make progress as you move through this program, and before you know it, you will come to realize that you are changing. Seeing this phenomenon for what it is (the mentality of a scared child being ruled by a dysregulated nervous system) allows you to mindfully and intentionally push past resistance to get into the groove of the work.

Let me share the motivational speech I give to my clients: We are talking about your life here. There is no room for sabotage. You have been standing still for too long. What we're discussing can help to protect you from yourself, and the most powerful weapon in your arsenal is knowledge. You now understand the process by which your protective and well-intentioned human brain creates physical pain to divert you from emotional injury. Allow this to empower you with the strength to push past your resistance and do the work.

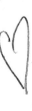

DENIAL OF THE SYNDROME IS PART OF THE SYNDROME

When explaining TMS, Dr. Sarno often said, "Denial of the syndrome is part of the syndrome." This means that your brain will invent creative ways to try to convince you that this work will get you nowhere. So let's debunk all of that right now. I am telling you straight up, this work will get you everywhere. It will *take* you everywhere. Resistance may whisper in your ear, "Nicole's combo of mindset, journaling, and being nice to myself is going to relieve chronic pain that no doctor could? It sounds too basic to be true." It's not. *The ability to express oneself without fear is transformative.* It literally rewires your brain. And that's where we are going.

A smart friend used to say to me, "Life is a behavior modification program." Despite your best efforts, you can't think your way into better feelings. Maybe you tried it last night from three to five a.m. rolling around in bed? Spoiler: It doesn't work. Any changes that may occur are always tied to action. And the small, measurable actions you take through mindset management and the practices you're learning here will help you overcome an enormity of pain and suffering. They will rid you of the false sense of control that your nervous system has been trying to provide you—and give you back your power, your health, and your life.

Let me take this opportunity to remind you: You are powerful. You have the agency to make a decision that serves your greatest good. It all starts here. So sit down, close your eyes, and decide:

I will do something hard.

I will do something uncomfortable.

I will take back my power.

I will allow in the light.

I will live the fullest, richest life available to me.

I will taste, touch, and feel everything.

I will no longer live a limited existence.

I am worth it, and I will begin today.

Make this decision, <u>recognize your resistance for what it is</u>, feel the love you have for yourself, and buckle up. We are on our way.

•

Sonja's Recovery from Complex Regional Pain Syndrome (CRPS)—Age 24 (Norway)

I thought I had pulled a muscle—I am a dancer and was stretching when I felt a sudden pain in my leg, so that was a logical conclusion. However, the injury did not heal. In retrospect, I now know there was never an injury. But it just kept getting worse, and some weeks later the same pain spread to my other leg as well. The pain became so bad that I couldn't walk anymore. I needed to quit dancing, halt my studies at university, and stop working at the pharmacy job that was supporting my schooling.

By this time I had seen three different doctors, and the diagnosis was still that I had a pulled muscle. Ridiculous, when I think of it now. How could an injury spread to the other leg and get so much worse over time? But doctors are "always right," so I thought, and I went home with painkillers and advice to rest.

For days I stayed home in bed, waiting for the pain to go away and the injury to heal. That did not happen. It just got worse and started spreading to other parts of my legs and upper body. I was getting depressed and really worried about what was going on. There was not a second in my day without pain. It was like being in a torture chamber—someone poking me with knives and burning objects *all the time.* Nothing helped. By the end of the year I had seen ten different doctors and three physiotherapists. I tried chiropractic, trigger point massage, different pain medications, diet changes, and supplements. All my medical tests were good, and according to doctors I was as healthy as can be. Yet I had this chronic pain.

The best time of the day was when the night came and I could sleep and feel no pain—except that by the fall of that year I was in pain even in my dreams. I couldn't cook, clean, or do anything physical. If I needed to walk to the bus stop that was one hundred meters from our door to go to the doctor, it took me twenty minutes to make it there. This, after being a dancer who could do complex routines for hours. I was twenty-five years old, but I felt like I was ninety-five.

The pain gradually spread all over my body and I was diagnosed with complex regional pain syndrome (CRPS), which has no cure. I couldn't even knit because the aching was also in my hands. I felt that I was a burden to my family; I was no joy to anyone. I hated life. I hated the pain. Nobody could help me, and I was all alone. I couldn't live like this anymore—not that you could call my life "living" at that point.

So I made a decision in November. I would give it one final chance: If I was not better by Christmas, I would end my life. As crazy as it sounds, I was happy about this decision. It gave me some peace: I would not need to be in agony much longer.

A couple weeks after that dark decision, I was scrolling online. I typed *Are there any people who have healed from chronic pain?* into the search bar. A video popped up. It was this nice lady, Nicole, explaining that chronic pain occurs because I do not feel my emotions.

She said if I learned how to journal in a specific way about all of these issues in my life, I could be totally pain-free. I can't explain to you why, but something woke up within me. Everything she said made perfect sense.

So I started JournalSpeak, twice a day, for twenty minutes. Nicole only insists you do it once a day, but I was on a mission. What came out was surprising; I hadn't known there were so many thoughts and emotions wanting to be heard! And the best part is that it really worked. Five days (just five days!) later, I could feel my pain levels starting to come down. The pain began to move around my body, and knowing that this was normal allowed my anxiety to ease.

I remember that my friend came over one day and I was able to make her a cup of tea and move around in the kitchen! It was like magic. It was hard to believe it was true. I was in heaven! After all these treatments and medications I had tried, all I had to do to heal was spend few moments of the day writing about my feelings on paper. How amazing is that? I know about the brain science now, and I realize it's not as simple as it felt in those early weeks, but I was so relieved that my life wasn't over, I could barely contain myself.

Two weeks into JournalSpeak, I was in my room looking out the window. It was a beautiful day, and the snowflakes were dancing in the wind. The whole year I had been watching people walk outside in the park from the little jail of my bed. That moment, the realization hit me: I could go outside and walk in the park! Nicole had taught me that nothing is dangerous about the way I feel—I experience the pain, but moving cannot hurt me. And so I put on my clothes and walked out onto the beautiful snowy road. I was so out of shape, but I didn't care. I'd thought I'd never walk like this again. It was wonderful. I think people take ordinary activities like walking for granted. They don't realize how blessed they are when they can do such things.

Slowly, very slowly, I got better. My pain moved all the time, though it mainly had a few favorite places in my legs. I learned through Nicole about the symptom imperative, and I finally understood why my pain has been morphing and changing all this time. Instead of being afraid or despairing, I got excited when the sensations would alter and shift. I had it on the run. I was on my way out of the woods.

Healing does not come easily. You need to do a lot of mental and emotional work for it to happen, but it's totally worth it. And you are going to get flare-ups. I had so many Mindbody issues during those years (heartburn, back pain, fatigue, sleep problems, anxiety, and depression). I just kept practicing acceptance and doing the work, knowing that the symptom imperative is not dangerous. It is simply a truth on this path to wellness.

My pain substantially descended from its peak, and I was able to start dancing again. I went back to university to finish my studies. Today I am able to do normal tasks with very little pain, and what's better, I no longer spend all my time in my bed! I play any sports I choose, and I dance both recreationally and competitively, which is so important to me. I know that my healing is a work in progress. I still JournalSpeak nearly every day. When I do have pain, which is minimal, I know it's because tuning down my overly kind and conscientious personality is hard. But I have tasted freedom from chronic pain, and I know this is my new normal.

Sometimes I have conflicting feelings that I don't know what to do with—kind of like a "404 page not found" situation. There is no instruction manual for my brain. Most of my conflict happens because the old me would have reacted differently than the person I am now. This is okay, though. Nicole always says, "Life is a choice between what hurts and what hurts worse," and I _know_ that being in chronic suffering is far more painful in every way.

The biggest challenge has been changing my mindset regarding myself: developing compassion, forgiveness, and acceptance. Replacing my negative self-talk with positive has made a huge difference. I am learning not to care so much about the good opinions of other people—and because of my upbringing, this has been a difficult task. I choose to think that I live in a friendly universe that wants only the best for me (which may not always mean fun or comfortable). I embrace the idea that all adversities and difficulties are here to offer a chance for growth and the opportunity to live a more fulfilling life in the future.

I am surprised how few people appreciate normal life and the beautiful moments it offers daily: the ability to move, do sports, or even go to the grocery store. To walk in the woods, to laugh with friends and family. I didn't laugh for almost a year! Or simply appreciating moments without pain. Just being without pain is something for which to be grateful. You can always find the gratitude if you choose to look for it.

I don't miss my formerly busy life with impossible schedules and too many things to do in a day. I'd been doing what I thought other people and society expected me to do, never considering why. This realization opened up a new freedom and a question: *What do I really want to do?* I feel that I am discovering the real person I truly am for the first time. It is a huge gift to get to know yourself.

CHAPTER 6

CREATING RITUAL AND CONSISTENCY

Many of the ingredients are in your mixing bowl: You've heard a little about my personal story (more to come), learned about the brain science, read about the mindset that calms your system, and looked resistance in the eye.

There's just one more thing we need to do before we can begin the work. And that's to develop best practices that will allow for the most powerful work.

It's time to talk about ritual and consistency.

Ritual and consistency give way to flow. We all know what it feels like to be in a state of flow. Problems seem to solve themselves. Answers come naturally without much fanfare. We also know what it feels like to be blocked and full of excuses. Personally, there is nothing that feels worse to me than the barrier of my own defiance. It shames me, depresses me, and paralyzes me. But, as we just hammered home for a whole chapter, it's important to remember that resistance thinks it's protecting you. So, no matter what, we meet it with self-compassion.

The gold at the end of the rainbow is an undeniable connection to intuition and presence (not to mention the cessation of chronic pain, illness, and anxiety), so let's finalize the road map that will bring you forward. Ritual and consistency are underrated. This is likely because they don't always come easily. Even so, we must fight for them. They create a structure around behaviors that serve our highest good, and they make it much more likely to achieve results. To motivate you when all the forms of resistance crop up, remember that you are (finally, at long last) partnering with yourself. This work has the power to forge, perhaps for the first time in your life, a healthy relationship *with you*. This is priceless, and as you experience it, you will begin to more readily make choices that support this beneficial alliance.

As you may recall from Chapter Four, much of our behavior is governed by habit. While we often discuss habits in terms of the ones we already have—and those we would like to break—it is essential here to build new routines that better support health and well-being. This takes time and effort, but it can be done.

Consider the example of adding exercise to your morning. Anyone who's set this kind of goal knows that it doesn't always come easily. Maybe you were full steam ahead about hitting the gym for the first day or two—perhaps it even lasted the week. But then comes the sunrise when you stayed up too late the night before. Or the morning when your favorite spin instructor isn't available. Perhaps your children or partner begin demanding your attention to address their needs. Or work has come calling with an unexpected deadline. Take your pick—there are millions of little distractions that might make it just that much easier to skip the gym.

But when you can override these diversions one by one, little by slowly, and continue showing up each morning, you will arrive at a habit. Most experts agree it takes about three weeks of consistent, repetitive action for this to happen. You arrive here by putting the right supports in place to make it (relatively) easy for you to attend your morning gym appointment day in and day out. With tenacity, you've found a way to build ritual and consistency.

The same is true for your JournalSpeak practice and meditative routine. As you prepare to start the work, it is imperative that we construct the pillars that will support you. Let's consider several key factors that contribute to best practices when it comes to doing this work.

PHYSICAL SPACE

It's remarkable how important physical space is. Everything has an energy to it. We too easily ignore the influence of a calm and safe vibe when attempting to try something new. When it comes to your JournalSpeak practice, choosing a physical space with the right energy for you is key. We are all different, and we find comfort in diverse environments. Sometimes the bustle and anonymity of a busy coffee shop with your headphones on is the perfect spot, or perhaps a shady bench in your neighborhood park feels good. Conversely, you might prefer the solace of your closet, your bedroom, or even your bathroom floor with the door locked (I've brought pillows in!). There are rooms to reserve in public libraries, the sanctuary of a car during lunch break, or a sign on your office door that says you'll be back in thirty minutes.

JournalSpeak can be accomplished with equal efficacy longhand or on a computer. Once again, personal preference will direct your choices. If a computer or tablet feels most comfortable, keep in mind that it will need to be charged, or your physical space should include a convenient outlet. These minor details may feel unimportant at the moment, but thinking ahead will prevent you from missing a session. This is especially crucial at the beginning of your journey when your nervous system needs a ton of consistency to settle into the posture of healing: rest and repair. Believe it or not, a dead computer on your lap in a park can feel like an overwhelming defeat. The lack of a pen when you've hidden yourself away in some little nook can seem like a sign to try again another day. Avoid situations like this by making every aspect of your practice a mindful act. Preparation is especially key for people with families or roommates. Open your mind and consider your possibilities.

In the end, the most important factor is finding a spot where you *feel free to feel*. This will sound like an alien concept to some. "Feeling free to feel" may be a notion you've never considered, but here it is essential. This writing is going to go deep, inviting you to release things in your reservoir that have the power to transform your physical body. The place where you will most readily accomplish this is the space that works.

TIMING

For me, this work is best endeavored in the morning before I lose the motivation to do it. I used to have a colleague who said, "I have to do anything difficult first thing, before I come to my senses!"

If morning is not a fit for you, because of schedule, family, or responsibilities, pick a time that feels right and stick with it. A lunch break works well, as does the creation of a bedtime ritual. Take an honest look at yourself. Do you operate best when the day is fresh, or does the hassle of morning override your ability to focus? Does in your car midday feel doable, or does an evening on the couch carry a sense of ease? It's not the time but the consistency that matters.

Scheduling can also be a factor if you are struggling to find physical space. For example, I know a lot of young mothers who choose to wake up thirty minutes early and do their JournalSpeak and meditation before their children rouse and wreak havoc on their morning routines. I know it's a bummer to steal from your precious sleep, but in the process of saving your own life there will be bummers. <u>Recall my constant refrain that life is a choice be-tween what hurts and what hurts worse. Choices must be made.</u> Perhaps hit the sack in the evening when your children go to bed, and then use the early morning for yourself.

Whenever possible, committing to the same time every day can be incredibly helpful in staying the course. If the word *commitment* sends a shiver of fear down your spine, welcome it with a grin. Yep, we hate that word. But it is necessary here. The sooner we accept that we need to have a faithful relationship with ourselves, the sooner that relationship can feel solid and safe. Like any partnership, not much is accomplished without the sense of security that commitment brings.

Sorry, not sorry: You and you are getting serious here. The essential message of the moment is that *you are important*. The priorities you set now will be the foundation of your wellness. Although your fearful and resistant mind may regularly suggest, "I'll do it tomorrow," I want you to keep in mind that the way you live today *is the way you live your life*. You need to start as you mean to go on. I have had to learn this lesson many times. When you make commitments to yourself and honor them, you build a life fortified with self-love and self-care. Oh yeah, and a life free from "chronic" anything.

BOUNDARIES

I'm going to go out on a limb here and suggest that the "you" in your life has fallen too low on the priority list. It's time for this to end. You deserve this work, and you are allowed to take time for yourself. Indeed, you must. The body will carry your stress until it has the permission and clear channel to release it. If tiny seeds of opposition are sprouting as we discuss physical space and timing, please allow a self-care mindset to sweep them away. This work is essential for your health, your growth, your peace, and your free-dom. You are no good to your partner, your children, your loved ones, your colleagues, or your friends if you are sidelined with chronic illness of any kind. It's time to stop being ashamed of put-ting yourself first.

Oh, the elusive boundaries. The B word. How we resist these fantastic friends! When I've discussed the importance of ritual and consistency with my clients over the years, they've come up with all kinds of reasons why they can't set boundaries. Here is a taste of these misconceptions:

I feel selfish.

I just can't.

People expect things from me.

This is the way I've always been.

People won't love me if I don't show up the way they want me to.

I will be shamed.

I will be shunned.

It's not "the right thing to do."

This is yet another form of resistance, and I need to be a little tough-lovey here. Remember our fave cliché: If you keep doing what you're doing, you'll keep getting what you're getting. To free yourself from the misguided protection of your own primitive system, you must draw boundaries with the people in your life who expect you to twist yourself into a pretzel to make them happy. I know that your children want you every second of the day, your partner prefers that you greet every request with enthusiasm, your boss "needs" you there early, your mother presumes that you will take that phone call, et cetera, et cetera.

These things may all be true, and they are also immaterial at the moment. You have the ability to change your life, and it's *your responsibility* to help others support you. You do this by enacting kind yet firm boundaries. You might say something with the energy of "I am choosing to do the work required to transform myself. As I heal, it will have a really positive influence on our relationship. While I'm doing this, I may need to take more personal time than you'd like. I also may need to ask for your patience as I manage the emotions that arise. Just like you are important to me, I know that I am important to you. I'm also realizing that I need to be important to me. I really appreciate your partnership in making this process possible for me."

One reason boundaries can be hard is that people in your life may feel threatened when you make room for yourself in a space they used to occupy. This can refer to literal space or "time space," during which you've typically cared for them. Remember, boundaries equal love. They not only support your growth but also teach other people how to treat you. In addition, they model, for your loved ones, how to honor themselves. Console yourself with these truths. If you see things in your relationships changing, consider that perhaps they needed to change. Often, in parenting my own children, I've mourned their "losses" when I've had to draw boundaries. Then, down the road, I discovered that those losses were exactly the ones they needed in order to grow. With loving, solid, and consistent boundaries, everybody wins.

I may have mentioned this before, but this is your *life*.

You are essential, incredible, beautiful, valuable, and unique. This time is for you, and you will never look back on it with regret. Over the years with clients, I've found that signing a contract can be a powerful symbol of commitment to this process. I've included one here with all of the points we've discussed. I invite you to sign it alongside a trusted witness and make a pledge to the future you absolutely deserve.

Now that we've laid the groundwork, it's time to get to the most powerful part—the transformation you've been promised. You've acknowledged your self-soothing strategies and the stories you've told yourself about your symptoms. You've set your expectations appropriately and are ready to address the ways you might resist this process. And now, you've taken a good, honest look at how to build ritual and consistency in order to make this practice a regular habit. You understand that you are precious and essential, and your boundaries will broadcast this lovingly to the ones who matter.

You are ready. It's time to do the work.

CONTRACT *(Have someone witness it, if it feels right!)*

I, _____, hereby commit to creating the kind of ritual and consistency in my life to support my Mindbody practices. Starting today, I am ready to partner with myself to take the time and space required to build a healthier relationship with me.

I will find a physical space where I feel free to feel. I will go there at a regularly scheduled time of day so I can make myself and my Mindbody work a priority. And I will set boundaries with those who mean the most to me so I can fully commit to my JournalSpeak practice.

I understand the power of ritual and consistency and its role in taking back control of my life and my chronic symptoms. I am important and I deserve this time and space to heal. I hereby pledge to make the changes necessary to build the future I deserve.

Love, me.　　　　　　*My witness:*

_____

Print Name　　　　　*Print Name*

_____

Sign Name　　　　　*Sign Name*

_____

Find your electronic copy of this contract at www.nicolesachs.com/contract.

●

Gary's Recovery from Chronic Fatigue Syndrome and Brain Fog—Age 62 (New Zealand)

I was diagnosed with chronic fatigue syndrome (CFS) after a viral infection. The day before I got sick, I had completed an eleven-hour hike through the mountains, so my level of fitness and general health were fine prior to being infected. For my age, they were excellent. I did not experience intense symptoms or need medical treatment during the initial illness. I had a fever and malaise, and generally felt unwell for a few days, but it wasn't worse than flus I have had previously. After a few days, I believed I had shaken it off, and I reentered life—albeit a bit limited on the physical side. Three weeks later I spent a long weekend on a planned hunting trip with friends, which included a lot of exertion. I could tell I was struggling. Something didn't feel right. This was the beginning of my decline.

Over the following few months, I recorded what was happening to me and tried many things to "beat" it. My primary symptoms were debilitating fatigue, brain fog, difficulty concentrating, breathlessness, and POTS (abnormally elevated heart rate). Some doctors labeled it long COVID. I found office work difficult and became mentally exhausted after short periods. Telephone calls left me breathless after ten minutes, and if I continued longer, I would have to lie down afterward to recover from the exertion.

I was reduced to walking small distances around the block. If I tried to lift anything or do any real kind of physical activity—however light—I would become immediately fatigued and have to lie down, possibly for hours. I also experienced post-exertional malaise (PEM), which triggered a "crash" the following day that at times affected me for weeks afterward. Talking to anyone wore me out. Just the thought of doing small things or having conversations left me drained. I learned that fatigue is "non-sleep-restorative," meaning I would arise feeling just as exhausted, even after a long sleep at night.

The cognitive demise was harder to measure, but I noticed I was becoming mentally exhausted and scattered after very small periods of concentration. I became unable to read or spend time on the Internet. After three months, I had to stop working as I was unable to concentrate at all, and I was making simple mistakes in important tasks. Especially terrifying, I was unable to locate the right words when talking to others, and I became breathless after just a few sentences.

A low point was when my son came back from university for a few days, and I was unable to have a conversation with him in spite of really wanting to. My world was becoming smaller and I had entered the "push and crash" cycle, wherein I would do something very insignificant, like climbing stairs, and pay for it for days or weeks afterward. I also noticed that when I was describing my symptoms to someone, or got in a negative thought pattern, I would feel worse.

Lying on a beanbag most of the day, unable to read or go online, became the norm. I was fearful of ending up bedbound, but that was looking like it could become a reality. I saw doctor after doctor. I tried supplements, anti-inflammatory diets, and other suggested life-style changes. All availed me nothing.

In spite of these warning signs, I had this underlying belief that nothing was wrong with me. Medical tests were all clear. A specialist suggested that my autonomic nervous system was stuck in the fight-or-flight setting, which satisfactorily explained the symptoms I was experiencing. This made sense, but what to do about it? During all this time, I was looking for possible solutions. The medical community had nothing to offer, and my own doctor admitted that they could only recommend rest and pacing. I was unable to read, so I resorted to YouTube videos as they required less effort. Even those were hard to concentrate on for long.

My wife began researching on my behalf, throwing herself into stories of long COVID recovery and other content on CFS. She found two sites with stories of individuals who had healed from similar situations. This gave me some hope, but it was also challenging to take it all in. I realized that I needed to improve cognitively to be able to help myself, so I reduced my life to a bare minimum. I moved to a camping ground to stay in our caravan for a while. I dedicated my energy to regaining my mind.

One term that kept coming up on the websites I clicked was *Mindbody*. I had no real understanding of what this meant, but I was determined to find out. I was lucky enough to read one recovery story of a woman named Esther that referenced a particular podcast. This podcast was an interview by Nicole Sachs with a woman named Lieke (I had never heard a podcast before).

Lieke had recovered from CFS and long COVID. I identified with her story and got a lot of hope from listening to that interview. During the podcast there was mention of more content I could find from Nicole.

Invigorated for the first time in a long while, I dove into more of what I could find of Nicole online. This was the major turning point for me. I needed to hear someone say "If you do X, you will get well." Not only did Nicole have this positive conviction, but she explained *exactly* what I needed to do. My biggest fear at the time was following the wrong approach to recovery. There were so many well-meaning but unfounded ideas out there, and I had such a minuscule amount of mental energy (concentration). I feared that if I invested in the wrong approach, I would remain unwell or even deteriorate.

I made a connection to my youth that helped me believe that what she suggested could be effective. As a child of seven or eight, I'd experienced migraine headaches at a certain time every Sunday. Even at that age, I hadn't believed they were caused by anything external. I'd felt I was somehow involved in their regular occurrence. Looking back and suspecting that perhaps something stressful had triggered those headaches helped me to believe that my current symptoms might also have an emotional origin. It wasn't difficult for me to then consider that the reverse might also apply—addressing my repressed emotions could alleviate my suffering.

I dedicated the coming weeks to healing myself following the instructions Nicole provided. Initially I journaled twice a day, followed by a period of calm breathing for twenty minutes. There is no doubt that I felt a little resistance at first—some symptoms intensified or swapped out for others and I was confused about what was going on. (I had yet to learn about the symptom imperative!) I found myself tempted to jump back into the medical model. However, each night as I lay in bed and took stock, I felt I was on the right track. I made a decision to trust the process completely.

A turning point came when I had the experience of a totally new symptom—a sharp pain in my back—and I was amazed when I was able to "turn it off" by saying or thinking the word *anxiety* and considering what was worrying me. Although I had yet to fully understand the brain science at this point, it reinforced that there was some link between what I was feeling and what I was experiencing physically. I now know that this intentional message sent a communication of safety to my nervous system, precluding the need for the symptom to continue.

As I went on, ritual and consistency were key for me. I did my JournalSpeak in the morning right after my waking routine, and I did it every day. The combined process of taking Nicole's course and consistently doing JournalSpeak enabled my full recovery. Nicole also emphasized kindness and compassion for myself, which was such a foreign concept to me that I had to Google what it meant!

Getting through difficult moments was made easier by paying attention to the fact that sometimes my symptoms "forgot" to appear. I was absolutely amazed. One morning I decided to grab my bike and see what I was capable of. Shockingly, I did three hours of bike riding and hill climbing with no consequence. This was incredible, given I had been rendered breathless by doing a few minutes of activity just weeks earlier. I had a flare-up of symptoms for a couple of days the following week, as my body made a last-ditch attempt to "protect" me, but by then I had hard evidence of this process curing me. They subsided quickly. While it took a little bit longer, my cognitive ability fully returned, and I was so grateful to have my mind back.

Everyone's recovery is different, but I want to say this because I feel like my consistency caused it to happen: Within two months of beginning this process I returned completely to normal activities, including traveling overseas. There is no timeline that is set in stone for recovery. My best advice is not to get caught up in worry, to set your ritual, and just to do the work. I am confident you'll see results.

I am forever changed in the way I view the human experience. I'm amazed at just how powerful we can be. Alongside my normal work and exercise routine, I have dedicated a portion of my life to helping others with CFS and long COVID in New Zealand and Australia. I reach out to people, share my story, and refer them to Nicole's teachings. To think I had never heard a podcast, and the first one I listened to saved my life.

HEAL: RETRAINING YOUR BRAIN

CHAPTER 7

UNDERSTANDING JOURNALSPEAK

N ow that we have laid the proper foundation for the journey ahead, it's time to delve into the brain-changing practice of JournalSpeak.

JournalSpeak is a daily form of expressive writing. So, yes, journaling. When I used to introduce JournalSpeak to my clients, there was often some initial cynicism. Journaling, in and of itself, is not a new tool. Many of them had tried some form of it before. And if they had, they wondered how writing things down was going to provide any relief for migraines or an IBS flare-up. I understand this suspicion all too well. It makes perfect sense, but in the end it's just another form of resistance. The best thing about having so many years of experience doing this work with people is that I know exactly when I need to protect you from yourself. No one can be helped when they are being bossed by their inner skeptic, so let's take a minute to break it down.

Before I tell you what JournalSpeak is, let me tell you what it is *not*. JournalSpeak is not jotting down notes about your day because you'd like to keep a record. This isn't a gratitude journal where you try to focus on the good to spiritually lift yourself out of whatever pain you're in. And JournalSpeak isn't just a free-writing exercise where you can ignore the uglier or more complex things that come up in response to a prompt.

JournalSpeak is a form of targeted self-expression specifically designed to get to the heart of your repressed emotions.

This vehicle gives you total permission to let your inner child speak—and release your feelings, no matter how ugly, angry, or inappropriate they may seem, before they threaten to overwhelm your emotional reservoir.

So while you may have been doing some kind of journaling for years, it is not the same as a JournalSpeak practice. Success in JournalSpeak requires you to come to it with the pointed understanding that your repressed emotions are directly connected to the physical pain or chronic symptoms you experience. You need to write in a way that invites your unconscious mind to know that it is safe for your overwhelming core feelings to surface—and your nervous system does not have to provide a headache or back pain to move you into rest-and-repair mode, engaging something you can "control."

Remember: Your brain thinks it's protecting you. The question is, from what? The answer is simpler than you realize. It is our un-thinkable, defiant, and conflictual thoughts and emotions. They threaten us somehow, and we "believe" that acknowledging and feeling them will kill us. This, of course, is not rooted in any truth—scientific or otherwise. As Dr. Sarno's groundbreaking work has shown us, the mind's desperation to protect us from these feelings is the direct cause of much chronic pain, muscle constriction, neuropathy, bodily inflammation, chronic anxiety, and more.

NOT ALL EMOTIONS ARE CREATED EQUAL

Let's talk emotions—a topic largely ignored or dismissed as unimportant in medical circles. As you are learning here, however, emotions are central to the messages of danger we inadvertently send our protective systems. Until we integrate this essential truth, it is nearly impossible to be chronically well.

Living within each of us are these *core feelings*: grief, despair, rage, shame, and terror. No one is immune. They are not polite, and they rarely feel appropriate to share in any context. We tamp them down and make way for more "socially acceptable" emotions we label with words like *regret, confusion, frustration, fear*, and *insecurity*.

As they are so off-putting (to both ourselves and others), we are far less likely to refer to these uncomfortable core feelings in casual conversation. While you might lament to a friend that you are "irritated" or "struggling," you are rarely willing to admit that you are "enraged" or in "despair." It's essential to know that these guttural emotions stir within every one of us and are perceived as acutely dangerous by your nervous system based on your unwillingness to look them in the face. They are connected to various stories, past trauma, relationships, and experiences that have hurt and shaped you. You may not even be *consciously* resistant to facing these paper tigers, but without awareness of their existence, your nervous system has no choice but to enact protection against them again and again.

Your core feelings stir beneath the surface of propriety. It feels "wrong" to say (or even think) it, but you resent your ailing parents for requiring so much of you. You hate your kids for their moodiness and entitlement. You loathe yourself for being less successful than you'd hoped. You harbor a growing grudge against your partner for not recognizing that you need them to do more around the

119

house. You are not just pissed off about the things that you're tasked to tolerate, *you are enraged*. You are not simply "freaked out" or worried. *You are terrified*. The problem is, depending on your upbringing and your nature, you may not even be conscious of these feelings. You may have difficulty detecting them or giving them a specific label. Instead, you just know that your back hurts, your head throbs, your skin itches, your stomach churns, or you lie awake anxious all night.

The reason that chronic pain and conditions have become such an epidemic is that these core feelings are *relentless in their reflex to rise*. You have no choice about this, no matter how "strong" you are. It doesn't matter how well-adjusted to modern life you believe yourself to be. These emotions demand to be felt—one way or another.

Envision a child playing with a beach ball in a pool. The goal of the game: Keep the ball underneath the water. The game ends as soon as the ball breaks the surface. I don't know if you've ever tried it, but holding a beach ball underwater takes a great deal of effort. The beach ball, in this metaphor, is those core feelings. Like the child desperate to keep the ball pushed down, our brains fight relentlessly to keep our negative feelings submerged and out of conscious reach. We "believe" that if they breach the surface of our awareness, we won't survive. This way of thinking takes so much energy—even if we are not always consciously aware of it.

The language of JournalSpeak translates your surface feelings, the ones you are actually aware of (pissed, worried, embarrassed), into the deeper, more unpleasant truths that must be acknowledged (enraged, panicked, ashamed) to eliminate chronic symptoms. Your body will stop sending messages of pain to your nerves and muscle groups once you've learned how to allow these "threatening" feelings to rise. Situations don't need to be rectified for this to happen— you just need to *know*. The goal of a JournalSpeak practice is to create a vehicle by which these submerged truths can find their way to consciousness safely. When this is difficult to believe, allow the stories within these pages to be your solace. Dip again into the brain science. This process has cured not only me but untold numbers of people.

Anyone can learn how to speak this transformative language. And, most importantly, you need only speak it to yourself. No one else needs to bear witness to the core feelings that reside within you—simply allowing the emotions to rise convinces your brain that you are safe. There may be some attendant suffering as these deeper feelings come to the surface, but you will not die. This is news to your nervous system, and that's why we must deliver it in a calm voice. Remarkably, not only will acknowledging your repressed emotions *not* kill you, you will thrive. Your body will not need to work so hard diverting you from experiencing them.

A NEW FORM OF EMOTIONAL EXCAVATION

I developed JournalSpeak at one of the lowest points in my life. Recovery is not a straight line, and my story has two acts. As I mentioned earlier, my mom (and Rosie O'Donnell) first introduced me to Dr. Sarno's work in my early twenties. After understanding the message of his incredible book *Healing Back Pain*, I accepted that repressed emotions were tied to my own struggle. If I acknowledged them without resistance, the pain signals would abate. And they did. I would learn years later, however, that recognizing the feelings and connecting them to my physical problems was not enough. I needed to dig deeper to change the ways in which my brain sought to protect me. Here's what went down.

Nearly a decade had passed since my introduction to Dr. Sarno. Mindbody theories had freed me from my diagnosis and its attendant "rules" on how I had to limit myself. I had built a life. I completed my master's degree in social work, got married, and had two full-term babies without a hint of the drama that the doctors of my teens had predicted. My back had left me in peace. Then, one spring afternoon, as I picked up my ten-month-old son, Oliver, in his baby walker, to move him to the driveway where he could toddle safely, I felt a searing, electric pain sweep across my lower back. It felt like someone had taken a hot knife and dragged it right through my vertebrae. To this day, I don't know how I managed not to drop the baby once that lightning bolt hit.

I hobbled into the house and lay down on my couch. All of my appreciation of the Mindbody connection vanished in that moment. Fear led the entire conversation. Anguish filled my consciousness. Guilt and shame at not having listened to the doctors' decrees swallowed me. I staggered anxiously back to traditional medicine, desperate to alleviate my agony.

I tell you this part of the story in the spirit of total partnership and common humanity. Every one of us is susceptible to regression when we are in abject terror. Every one of us is vulnerable to the protection of our thoughts, their only goal being to save our asses. Forgive yourself for your backslides. Forgive yourself for your doubt. You can only do the best you can do in the moment, and in this moment, this was my best.

Over the course of several months, I spiraled. I was in physical therapy three days a week. I received "electric stim" treatments, therapeutic massages, and steroid shots. While some of these therapies helped for a bit, the pain always came back—sometimes worse. My doctors prescribed opioid medications and muscle relaxers. I took benzodiazepines to help me sleep. The pain was keeping me from embracing life. I was a detached partner and, although I am ashamed to admit it, an impatient and unkind parent. I felt so lost. It was a dark, vulnerable time.

As I rounded out a year of this hell, I found myself one late afternoon in a neighborhood deli with my kids, ages one and three. While I tried to pay for our food at the counter, my children did what most toddlers do—they started to run amok. They were grabbing containers of gummy bears and yogurt-covered pretzels. They were laughing, squealing, and full of enthusiasm for this activity. You know how they kindly call kids "spirited" when they're being total assholes? Well, mine were fully in the spirit on this particular day. I was trying to give my credit card to the cashier while awkwardly grabbing random containers out of their hands before the lids popped off and made a mess all over the floor. As soon as I wrenched one away from each of the little monsters, the other picked up something else. Although I know this scene is far too relatable for any parent, in the moment, I was more than a little overwhelmed and embarrassed. It seemed like everyone was looking at me—and I felt like the worst mother.

Somehow, I managed to pay and corral my kids so we could leave. I had each by the wrist so no one could wriggle free in the busy parking lot. I also had our purchases and a heavy diaper bag slung over my shoulder. As we approached the car, I felt my back start to tense up. I knew this feeling all too well. I could already anticipate the searing, electric pain that was coming my way. I froze, knowing that if I moved any further, I could throw my back out.

I stood at the driver's side of my car, but I couldn't reach for my keys and keep a hold on each child as traffic whizzed by. I didn't have the mobility to do both. I couldn't open the door. I couldn't get my kids safely into their car seats. I was absolutely stuck. I don't know how long we stood there. I just rested my forehead on the window and sobbed. My kids, understanding that something was really, really wrong, stopped wriggling. They stood there, just looking up at me as I fell apart, making me feel even more broken and ashamed.

I'm not sure how I managed to hoist everyone into the car, let alone get us home. I somehow bathed my kids and put them to bed. I hobbled into the sanctuary of my room and sat down on the bed. I looked out the window and stared into the expanse, the trees and the stars. And in that moment, I surrendered. Enough was enough. This pain was no longer just torturing me, it was endangering my children. If it wasn't something I could get rid of with all the physical therapy, massage, treatments, medication, and rest I had been trying, I needed to do something different. I remembered Dr. Sarno. I remembered the cosmic shift that had defined my life after understanding the mind-body connection, and in that moment, I knew I needed to see him in person. My body was in rebellion, and nothing traditional was working. I was done complying.

I made an appointment. Before traveling to New York City, I sat down and wrote an entire novel about my experience with back pain, chronicling the date of every flare-up since adolescence. I noted what hurt and when; I delineated each body part and its attendant sensation. I outlined all physical activity and the agony attached to every bend, stretch, and effort. As I walked into the office, I solemnly handed this pain autobiography to Dr. Sarno, announcing its relevance. He took the pages from me—and there were so many pages!—and, while kindly looking me in the eye, dropped it into the metal garbage can next to his desk. It landed with a loud clang.

"This isn't important," he told me. "I don't need to know every detail and drama." I was mildly offended, yet tentatively hopeful. He had my attention. I love the confidence of a person who knows more than I do. He continued in his characteristic dryness, "Let's examine you and see what we find."

He gave me a thorough physical examination. He looked carefully at all of my films. And then, without production or spectacle, he told me that nothing was wrong with me.

"Your pain is due to tension myoneural syndrome, TMS," he said.

He went on. "Yes, you have a structural finding. These doctors are not incorrect. But spondylolisthesis does not cause pain. Neither does a bulging disc. They are thought to be the reasons for suffering, but this is not true." (The man was cool as a cucumber while delivering this message, almost like it was boring to him.) "You have what I like to call a normal abnormality, and there's nothing wrong with you that some emotional excavation can't fix."

I was relieved, but this was not yet a celebration on any level. "Okay, then," I begged, "but what do I *do*?"

Dr. Sarno spoke of the "reservoir of rage" inside each and every one of us. I began to gather that the notion of this reservoir is often alluded to in casual conversation. Think "I'm going to boil over any second now!" Or, "I'm going to blow my top!"

My overflowing reservoir of rage? I thought. This man was certainly on psychedelics. I was the least angry person I knew. I was so upbeat and lovely! I always helped everyone and rarely even expected my own needs to be met. Anger? C'mon. Rage? No way. He clearly was not getting me. "Dr. Sarno," I offered gently, "I'm not an angry person. Maybe I've got something going on in there, but it's not that."

"Oh, you're angry all right!" He laughed out loud, which was kind of embarrassing but, I have to admit, also revealing. "You're just feeling it through your back."

Dr. Sarno told me there was a way to end this cycle. I needed to address the connection between my anger and my pain. I had to find a way to allow my repressed emotions to safely rise. He told me that the most effective way to achieve this was through journaling, and he suggested that I write about how I was feeling for thirty minutes every morning and thirty minutes every night. I should begin, he said, by making three lists: one for childhood (or past stressors), one for daily life, and one for personality. Dr. Sarno explained that there was a certain set of personality traits that contributed most to chronic pain and the need to shove down our feelings—things like people-pleasing, self-criticism, and an overwhelming need to be seen as "good." The lists were a bulleted-out inventory of anything that might be causing me anger or anxiety—and then I was to write about them as needed during those two time slots.

All righty, then. One thing you should know about me: I am one of those type A students. I love to get a teacher's instructions and not only follow them to the letter but then add in just a little bit extra. I now know with a gentle laugh that this character trait is part of the reason I suffered in the first place.

So I made my lists. They were pretty long. I moved through them, detailing difficult memories, inventorying daily life and its annoyances, admitting challenging characteristics that colored the way I met the world. Nothing felt revelatory, but I was a rule follower and I was doing what I was told.

I found myself avoiding one bullet under *daily life*: *Motherhood*. The voice in my head said, *Skip that one, you know how you feel! Obviously. Everyone knows. It's wonderful and tiring. Heartful and hard. No need to linger there.* But there was a graver and persistent urging that kept bringing my eyes to that line on the paper. *Motherhood.* I scrawled it on the top of the page, and I began to write.

At first, I was transcribing what you might expect from a mother of two kids in diapers: *It's hard to be a mom. I never know if I'm doing it right. I'm really tired all the time. I wish I had more help.*

But then my writing took me to an unexpected place. As I read over the words on the page, I felt uneasy. *You're lying*, an inner voice said. I knew I wasn't *actually* lying, but I couldn't help but acknowledge that I was not excavating the truths that had the power to banish my back pain. My words were insufficient. I needed to be braver. I took a deep breath, looked down at the page, and then penned the first-ever line of JournalSpeak:

I hate being a mother.

I stared blankly, shocked by the words on the page. Those who know me understand that I have always yearned to be a mom. I was clear in my desire to have a family since I was ten years old. I spent years tormented, having been told I wouldn't have biological children thanks to my spondylolisthesis diagnosis. I had overcome everything and everyone to have my two precious babies. Yet.

Somewhere along the way, in the most natural and human way possible, I had become toxic with the striking and unrealistic expectations about what motherhood would be like.

As any parent or caregiver knows, the day-to-day life of parenting is anything but rosy. It's a hot mess. Although I was able to recognize and even vent about this, the unconscious grief and rage bubbling under the surface were aching to break free. The more inconvenient truths began to rise—*I need my children to be perfect to reverse the pain of my own childhood. I need the parenting experience to repair what I feel is broken inside me.* These revealing admissions were not at all available to me prior to this fateful day, but as they knocked on the door, I opened it with the desperation only the dying can appreciate. And many of us are dying in these moments.

My pain had been screaming for me to listen. To start, I had to confess that being a parent wasn't meeting the expectations I had created in my head. I had to confess, in that moment, that I hated being a mom. *Hated it.* I hated what it had done to my life, and how I was at the beck and call of my toddlers. I worried it would limit my potential—that I'd remain this tired and overwhelmed forever. I was scared that it would never get better. And each and every one of these feelings demanded to be felt.

This is the core power of JournalSpeak: The words are only true until your repressed thoughts and emotions are allowed to rise and be acknowledged. As soon as I put that deep, scary, and visceral truth on the page, I realized that I didn't hate being a mother. I loved my babies—I loved my family. Hmmm, then what was *true*?

I kept writing. I started to delve deeper to explore what might be leading me to have such strong negative emotions about parenting. I asked myself hard questions. I had to know what was driving the feelings of rage, shame, and despair. I realized that when I was a child and felt sad or alone, I made a subconscious plan to make things better. My eleven-year-old self's strategy for combating scary feelings was to tell herself that she would make her own family one day—and it would be *perfect*. It would erase all the pain she'd had to endure as a child. Having my own family, my *impeccable* family, would make me complete. I would be safe and whole.

I was waking up, more every second. I stopped being afraid of the unpleasant thoughts that were jumping into view, one after another. Instead, I became curious—*What else is in there?* I wrote and wrote, and my JournalSpeak began to span the length of my experience, inviting me into unexplored places in my heart and memory. I went back to the wounds of my upbringing; I looked my abusers straight in the eye and told them what they did to me. I stood up for myself. I fell to my proverbial knees and asked forgiveness with humility only accessible when no one is looking. I cried and protested. I let my inner child take the stage and be heard. I invited all of my demons to the kindergarten carpet, and I made space for everyone to have their say. I hated and loved, both others and myself. I set myself free.

Being able to be that honest, to understand where my parenting expectations came from, was transformative. It allowed me to lower the levels of my emotional reservoir and, in the process, completely eliminated my back pain.

It became a practice. I named it JournalSpeak, and for a long while I did it every day. I continued to uncover the things I was angry about. But as my proficiency in this type of excavation grew, I realized that my pain didn't only stem from rage. There were other core emotions demanding to be reckoned. Soon I expanded Dr. Sarno's "reservoir of rage" to include all of the extreme feelings: terror, grief, despair, shame, anguish, and many others that we normally fail to address. These feelings are not socially acceptable, so you keep them locked down deep inside. As we discussed earlier, while you can easily tell someone you are "stressed out," you rarely express that you are feeling despair, anguish, or shame. You certainly can't tell people that you hate being a parent.

I was healing, and I was changing the rules. I realized that if the brain perceives my repressed emotions as a greater predator than my physical pain, I need to address *all of them*, air them in the light. JournalSpeak provided a way for me to safely and methodically examine these core feelings. The pain was no longer necessary. It lost its reason for being.

My success led me to return to Dr. Sarno's office and share my approach. We spent hours talking about the ways in which I was integrating his work with clients in psychotherapy, and he began to refer patients into my practice. He suggested that my methods required a bigger stage and asked me to start lecturing with him on his monthly alumni panel in New York City. I shared my story and the process of JournalSpeak with others who were looking for ways to bring their unconscious emotions to the surface. This was just the beginning, and the reason we sit here together today.

I can understand if you still harbor some skepticism. Many of my clients did before they started the work in earnest. But if you open your mind and gently invite these daunting core feelings to rise in your JournalSpeak, you can transform your life. It is real, it is powerful, and it will send your pain on its way.

•

Charlotte's Recovery from Severe Foot Pain/ Swelling Due to Accessory Navicular Bone— Age 16 (Mid-Atlantic United States)

I was ten years old when I got my first pointe shoes. The director of my studio surprised me with the news after class one day as I got into my mother's car. I burst into tears. I was so excited. Getting *en pointe* is a huge deal for classical ballet dancers, and dance was my passion. At the time I was taking three ballet classes a week, in addition to jazz, contemporary, and lyrical dance. There was nothing more important to me.

Ten was a year earlier than was recommended for pointe in the dance world, but I was advanced for my age. I took class with girls a year older than me, and I couldn't wait to move into their ranks. My mom was a little concerned that it was unhealthy for growing feet to start so young, but she'd never have stood in my way. I did, however, know how she felt. I recognized that ballet is hard on a dancer's body, especially their feet.

Months passed, and I turned eleven. I was excelling at dance and loving the way pointe expanded my ability to thrive. One day I came home from class and showed my mother a bump on my feet that I'd never noticed before. It was a protrusion right below each ankle, as if I had a second ankle on each foot. The bones were a touch red and inflamed, and ached a bit but not terribly. My mom exclaimed, "Oh my God, do you think this is from the pointe shoes? We shouldn't have gotten them so young!" Even the great Nicole Sachs can be a hysterical parent.

We called and asked my studio director if she'd ever seen this, and we got some unexpected news. This was indeed something she'd witnessed before—she even had it herself. It was called an accessory navicular bone and affected about fourteen percent of the population. In most people it was no problem and asymptomatic. But, she said, in dancers it *could* create an issue because the bones might become inflamed with habitual wear and tear. She advised us to see an orthopedist.

As you probably know by now, my mom is a Mindbody practitioner and expert on chronic pain, but she has never failed to access the medical model when we are sick or hurting. It's the first step. And she can get scared when something might be wrong with her child. We made the doctor's appointment, and as the days passed, my "extra ankle bone" swelled and the pain worsened. At one point it was bright red and throbbing, like a golf ball.

At the doctor's appointment, stuff really got dark. He examined me and took X-rays, and he was even more reactive than my mom and me combined. "This is one of the worst cases I've ever seen of accessory navicular bone!" he said. "This will almost definitely require surgery."

I was in tears. My mom sat there, quiet and concerned. We left the office and she reassured me that everything would be okay. She would look into what this meant for me. It would never stop me from dancing, she promised. I wasn't so sure. That doctor seemed pretty adamant.

I know now that this was really hard for my mom, as it would be for any parent. You want to do what's best and necessary for your kid, but in my mother's case, it was not a clear choice. She knew that TMS can cause any number of reactions in the body, and there isn't always a rhyme or reason for the way it shows up. She did exhaustive research on my condition. She confirmed that most people who have it are asymptomatic. In reading up on the surgery, she came upon a post by a dancer, only seventeen years old. She had the same diagnosis as me, had the surgery, and a year later the pain had not abated. Now she had more complex pain. There was neuropathy at the incision site. She had to quit dancing.

My mother came into my room. She looked at the red, inflamed protrusions on my feet, and she said the thing that ended up changing my life as a dancer (and as a human). She said, "You know what I do for work, right? <u>You know how sometimes people have big feelings they don't understand, and that the body can feel those feelings for them physically?</u>" I did know. I had heard her talk about it many times. But it never occurred to me that *my body* might do that.

She explained to me that she had been worried, but now she wanted to treat my pain as TMS. She told me about the dancer, and her neuropathy, and that it didn't sound like this surgery took away people's pain. She also told me that if fourteen percent of the population had this condition, there would certainly be dancers thriving despite it. Then she did something that I know she does for so many people out there—she told me calmly and confidently that this work would make my pain go away completely. She reminded me that she had had the same experience when she was young with a structural finding that was never the reason for her pain. We just needed to *do the work*, together. I believed her.

We sat down and made a list. She asked me to tell her all the things that could be making me worried, angry, sad, and scared. It wasn't easy. But there was nothing that was going to stand in the way of dancing, so I complied. We talked about school and my extreme perfectionism that had been torturing me since I could remember. We talked about my friends—one in particular—who made me ragefully angry. We talked until we covered as many topics as we could think of, and I knew what she wanted me to do—get it *out*. I sat in my bed with a notebook and I wrote about the things that felt the most emotional in whatever way an eleven-year-old could. I have little recollection about what they were, but I know one thing—I got better.

Little by little at first, and then kind of all at once, the pain went away. The swelling would come and go, and my mom made a point to get me ice packs for my ankles. I know why she did it now. She wanted me to have a solid thing to feel control over. I could get the packs out of the freezer and bring them in the car on the way to dance. I could tell she thought I didn't need them, and secretly I agreed with her, but it felt good that I had a tangible thing to soothe me. Then one day I forgot to grab the ice packs, and another day. I barely noticed when we both forgot long enough to forget forever. I was symptom-free. Aside from the structural protrusion from the extra bone, my feet looked totally normal. They never even swelled again.

The years that followed brought Achilles tendinitis when I tried lacrosse, significant anxiety when I started middle school, and agonizing piriformis pain before a particular *Nutcracker* audition. Although these situations ranged from annoying to really upsetting, I never thought anything was wrong with me. I knew what to do. My mother would tell me kindly to do my JournalSpeak. I might storm to my room and give her the finger from behind my door, but I did it.

Today, I am sixteen and dance classical ballet over twenty hours a week. I am as passionate and dedicated to my craft as ever. I even had the incredible opportunity to share the stage with dancers such as Tiler Peck, Lucia Connolly, and Lyrica Woodruff during this season's *Nutcracker* performance. In addition, every summer I dance for weeks on end at ballet intensives, and never have I felt a tinge of pain in my accessory navicular bones. When my mom told me she was sharing stories, I insisted she share mine. I want to inspire people my age. It may be hard to believe, but it's honestly incredible the way our repressed emotions can cause pain in our bodies, even when doctors believe something is physically wrong with you. No matter how young or old you are, you can do this work. You have the power to help your body heal itself.

CHAPTER 8

JOURNALSPEAK AND MEDITATION ARE YOUR VEHICLES TO FREEDOM

I t's time to do this for yourself. Remember, our goal is to allow all of your core emotions—your rage, shame, despair, grief, fear, et cetera—to surface, bringing your emotional reservoir down to a manageable level. This will stop it from triggering pain. The good news is that, unlike Dr. Sarno's recommendation to journal twice a day for a half hour—who has time for that?—you can get this work done in a single thirty-minute session each day: twenty minutes of JournalSpeak followed by ten minutes of self-affirming meditation.

Many people have asked me over the years, "Can I do *more*?" Man, I love my type A babies. Yes, love, you can do more. But in my years of working with clients, I have found that twenty minutes of JournalSpeak is a sweet spot—a place where there is enough room for deeper truths to arise without hijacking your day or allowing your resistance to shut you down. If, like me at my lowest, you want to go ham and journal for hours, go to it. Just know that this is not imperative to heal. We need this process to be manageable and reasonable to your tantruming mind.

It may feel too good to be true that a practice like Journal-Speak can lead to such remarkable changes in your health and well-being—but paired with the mindset we've laid out here together, it can and does. I must remind you, however, that while this practice is simple, it is far from easy. It is going to require that you dig deep, unearthing painful feelings that your nervous system has deemed predators best kept at bay. The things that come up may surprise you—and it's best to be prepared for that. But life is a choice between what hurts and what hurts worse. As you move forward and become more proficient in JournalSpeak, you will soon see that the results are more than worth the effort and attendant discomfort.

In the pages that follow, we will delineate the specifics of an impactful excavation. At this point in the process, you may feel ready to embrace the practice but unsure where to begin—or whether you are doing it "correctly." As you make JournalSpeak part of your routine, you will find what works for you. In the meantime, I can offer a single response to the question, "How do I know if I'm doing it right?"

The only way to do it wrong is not to do it. So let's do it.

START AT THE BEGINNING

The translation of your surface truths into JournalSpeak begins by looking closely at your own story. When you thoroughly explore your life and experiences, your core truths will rise as your nervous system deems them safe, and it will no longer need to plague you with chronic pain. You can relax into the peace that is possible in your life.

At first, however, you just have to prepare for it to suck a little. You will not hate it every time you sit down to write, and this will not end you. But, as you've heard before, we need to set your expectations properly. If this were easy, there would be no rush on the brain's part to flood you with chronic suffering to help you avoid it. This is the hard stuff, the messy stuff. But it is also the beautiful, stunning, incredible, alive stuff that is going to set you free.

Your JournalSpeak practice starts with Dr. Sarno's recommendation to make lists for each of the three key categories: Childhood (or Past Stressors), Daily Life, and Personality. The Childhood list should comprise each event or relationship in your childhood or past from which you remember sadness, pain, conflict, or trauma. We all have our stories. When we tell them over and over to ourselves and others, I call it "playing our tapes." Human beings do this a lot, and it's a fine place to begin.

In a bulleted fashion, note the highlight reel of growing up. These bullets don't need to make sense to anyone else but you. If *Thanksgiving 1996* is enough to pull up an upsetting or profound memory for you, then that's one for the list. Bullets can also be vague if they are powerful to you. For example, my family moved and I changed schools a lot, and this gave rise to many issues with which I struggled for years. So *moving* stood as one item on my childhood list.

Under Daily Life, list the day-to-day dealings that stress you enough to notice, whether they involve work, family responsibilities, friendships, your annoying neighbor, or the irritating event that happened last week at the grocery store. Make line items for every member of your family and every significant person with whom you regularly share your life. Conflict is what creates big emotions, and our closest humans create our greatest conflicts. Overarching issues apply here as well. For instance, if *money* appears on your Childhood list because it was a concern growing up, also include it under Daily Life if it remains a source of tension. You'll find that although different items may cross lists, they often mean something unique in each context. This variation is good, as it gives you fodder for a more robust practice.

In my experience with clients, the Personality list can be a little harder to put together. Human beings are in a constant struggle between authenticity and attachment. This means that who you are and how you feel, deep down inside, can often conflict with what your family, workplace, and partner expect of you. This list should embody those conflicts—the self you feel pressured to present to the world that may torture you in your private moments. We are each born with a certain temperament, and our personalities are created by the ways in which our childhood experiences combine with that nature. This creates a lens through which you view the world.

Our personalities inform everything we do. In the Personality column, you might bullet out things like *I need to be well-liked by everyone* or *I feel uncomfortable and inadequate,* or *I need to please everyone all the time, even if I am the only one left hurting,* or *I am so threatened by conflict that I just give in . . . it's easier.* The biggest and hardest one for me personally was *I need to be perfect. If I can't be perfect, I may as well not be at all.* These longer sentences for traits like *people pleaser, perfectionist,* and *codependent* allow for an easier transition into JournalSpeaking about them.

No one is looking at these lists but you, so reach far and wide, and don't be afraid to include anything and everything that occurs to you. Here is an excerpt from my initial lists:

CHILDHOOD	DAILY LIFE	PERSONALITY
The time with the essay (6th grade).	Motherhood—two babies and tired/ spent.	I need to do everything perfectly, or I'm a failure (perfectionist).
The dinner at my cousin's sweet 16.	Marriage—feeling alone.	I'm not comfortable unless everyone likes me all the time.
Moving.	No job, no purpose.	I want to please everyone (people pleaser).
Dad helping me with HW.	Money.	I don't like to be in places with people who all know each other, and I'm the odd one out.
Mom and Dad's second separation.	My friend [name of person] and the way she makes me feel bad.	I feel alone even in a crowded room.
My first new bicycle (3rd grade).	Why is everyone always okay, and I'm not?	I never feel proud of myself even when I "know" I should be.

Find your electronic copy of this chart at www.nicolesachs.com/mylists.

This effort is just a starting point. As you get more experience with this work, your lists may evolve. Just make sure you are jotting down the things that speak to painful core feelings like shame, rage, terror, or despair. And make sure you're not consciously hiding from anything. When you get that squirrelly feeling that you'd prefer not to think about something because "What's the use? There's no changing it!" go right to it in your JournalSpeak practice. As I may have mentioned, we are saving your life here, and it's time to be done with the hiding.

I didn't realize early in my recovery that the "tapes" that inspired the items on my list weren't the whole story of what I needed to acknowledge to heal, but they were imperative to begin the excavation that would lead me to them. Think of your conscious issues on the lists, your surface truths, as the end of a pirate's treasure map—the X that marks the spot. Once each location is revealed, it's time to do the most important task. *You have to dig.*

The goal is to examine each item on your list. JournalSpeak about it until your symptoms begin to subside, and then continue to do so until the chronic pain, anxiety, spasm, inflammation, et cetera resolve. Be thorough, and never dismiss anything for appearing unimportant. Also remember that the nervous system's primary purpose is to keep you alive. Depending on the level of trauma or length of time you've been pushing things down, it may take a while to feel safe enough to release your pain. Please don't allow this to worry you. Recall that if it took twenty years to walk into the woods, you will not walk out in a few weeks. Putting a timeline on healing is another form of resistance. It can create more anxiety and urgency that leave your emotional reservoir at the tipping point. Instead of worrying about whether it's working fast enough, try to relax into the practice, knowing that you will feel what needs to be felt as you are ready. If you stick with the practice consistently, you will feel a shift.

WRITE IT OUT

Set aside thirty minutes a day for Mindbody work. The first twenty are for JournalSpeak.

Twenty minutes is long enough for the work to have impact and short enough for you to get on with your day. It's the right amount of time to dig in, but it's not so much time that you'll find it unmanageable. You can do this.

So set your timer for twenty minutes, take a bullet point from one of your three lists in whichever order you'd like, put it at the top of the page, and begin to explore how you feel about it. If you are unsure what to pick, take a breath and just consider your items. Which of them is calling to you? Is there something that is demanding to be felt? Or perhaps there's one you keep skipping over. The red flag is flying in your face. Pick that one.

Once you've selected the topic, open your mind, and free-write as best you can. Use *all* your language—and don't be afraid to be impolite. This is the time for you to let your inner child scream if they need to. *"Fuck them!" "I hate you." "I'm leaving and never coming back!" "I'm so sad I'll never stop crying." "I can't do this." "I will never feel better."* You are forgiven for anything you need to say when you are JournalSpeaking. These words are essential in lowering the level of your emotional reservoir—they are teaching your nervous system that you are safe to feel.

The first ideas to arise as you are writing will be your surface truths. Remember, these feelings are real, but they may not be the more revealing truths that must come out to alleviate your pain. Yet you must start somewhere, and this is a great place to start. Storytell. Say what happened and when. Don't be afraid to begin with simple anecdotes. Be a court reporter and state the facts. The big stuff will come knocking when it's ready.

Journaling your way out of pain will look different from other types of venting you've done in the past. Once you master the art of JournalSpeak, your writing will reveal hidden places in your recollections that need to be reckoned with. This process may involve bravely seeing your part in what has happened to you or allowing yourself to feel the spectrum of emotions that accompany certain memories or events—even when it is inconvenient to feel them.

Try not to become defensive. I know it wasn't your fault that you were abused or neglected. You were just a child. But here's the thing—the child sometimes *does* think it's their fault, and it's that child we are finally ready to hear. One of my greatest sources of release was the day I cried in my JournalSpeak, begging my dead father to forgive me for being such a disappointment. Of course, as a sentient adult I know that this is preposterous. It was not my job as a child to make a grown man feel good about himself. But if we needed only to hear from the version of me today, we would never be here in the first place. The little kid left behind in the wake of surviving childhood is the one who needs a voice now. Don't let your reflexive self-protection block its powerful, healing force.

As you move through the beginning phases of this work, remind yourself over and over that the truth will not end you, it will set you free. Talk to that sweet nervous system of yours. This may feel counterintuitive at first and, admittedly, it requires a bit of faith in the process. As your body becomes your proof, however, you will see the method to the madness. Remember also that no matter what arises for you, *you do not need to change your life in any way to be free of pain.* When I spoke to audiences with Dr. Sarno at NYU Medical Center back in the day, this was the most frequent query: "But I can't quit my job! Leave my marriage! Abandon my kids! Rob a bank! How do you propose I release this pain and anxiety without removing my life's stressors?"

We would explain: You need only consciously *feel* the spectrum of your core feelings. The pain is here to divert and protect you from that which the brain and nervous system deem a survival threat. We may not be able to solve all your problems, but we *can* get you out of pain. Becoming bilingual in your native tongue and JournalSpeak will hand you back your life. Your problems may not disappear, but you will be better equipped to meet them with grace. It is astonishing to see what transpires when you're not spending all of your energy keeping the proverbial beach ball under the water.

As you move through your lists, you may be wondering how to most adeptly undertake this excavation process. I understand. It doesn't necessarily come naturally. In my years of working with clients as well as embracing this practice myself, I've seen many examples of productive JournalSpeak. I think the best way to illustrate this new language is to give you a sample translation. Here is an adapted version of a surface truth (a quick playing of the tapes). It is not derived from one person but is instead an amalgamation of many stories I've heard and witnessed, including my own:

Bullet Point: My Affair

I am cheating on my husband. I don't know what I'm doing. I don't even know what matters to me anymore. I mean, my kids will be fine. They are teenagers, they don't even care what goes on with my husband and me. They are so self-absorbed. And you know, I'm not even that upset about it, because the truth is that he has been absent for years. He doesn't pay attention to me at all. My friends know me better than he does. I used to care, but I don't even think about it that much anymore. I don't know if I want to leave or not. I don't know what to do . . .

Now, with that surface truth revealed, let's invite the writer to take a breath and consider that she need only speak the truth to herself. She can own her part, her feelings, her role, and her power. Let's give this sharing another go in JournalSpeak:

Bullet Point: My Affair

I'm cheating on my husband. I know exactly what I'm doing. I'm finally, at long last, doing what the hell I want to do. That asshole has tried to control me and tell me how to feel since the day I met him, and honestly . . . I've had it. I'm fucking angry.

Why am I so incredibly angry? I can try to bullshit myself, but I know the truth. I'm angry at myself for being so stupid to think that a person would change completely just because he went from a boyfriend to a husband. I knew who he was when I married him. He showed me all the time! I chose to ignore it. I have no idea why. Yes, I do. No, I don't. Ugh. I hate myself for this kind of uncertainty! I feel like maybe I created this? I asked for it? I feel scared when I feel unsure . . .

Somehow, all of a sudden, I feel angry at my parents, especially my mother. I never say this out loud, but why did they make so many selfish choices? They created a child who was so desperate for stability and love that she would sacrifice her own self-esteem for what looked good on paper!

I wish I had the courage to talk about all of this. I am so insecure. I think I know why I'm so conflicted about everything all the time: I don't even know if I actually remember enough of my childhood to believe myself.

I'm so sad. I'm sad when I think about that girl . . . that little girl who was me. I'm so sad for that child, who thought she had the answer to the dilemma of a family who made her feel less than. She was so naive. I cry for her innocence. She had such a strong notion that she could repair it all with the perfect family that she had the power to create when she grew up. That sweet girl used her idealistic imagination to deny all of the warning signs. My God . . . she didn't even allow herself to have a clue that any of these truths existed!

She was me. She is me.

I am a mother and a wife, but this is not what I expected at all. I have no idea what I expected, but I do know that it was so fucking stupid like the old movies I used to watch with my grandma. My grandma was nice to me, actually. I remember that. I miss her. Since she passed away, I never allow myself to really think about that. I don't want to feel sadder than I already am.

You know what, though? I'm a grown-up now, and if I am brave enough to speak it, I think I actually know what matters to me. I'm not usually comfortable saying it out loud, but I think I kinda know.

I want a partner to raise kids with, not just a placeholder. I want to be a good Mama, still, even though they don't call me that anymore. I want to be acknowledged! I want to be appreciated. I want to be heard. Inside, I feel like I want to scream . . . pretty much all the time.

I know what I did. Instead of asking for any of these things in an understandable manner, I just drifted away. I became a cheater, something I swore was beneath me. I can't justify it. I feel like a disgusting failure. I'm sick over it. And you know what's worse? I'm so scared that my kids will be fucked up forever.

I know they are watching every interaction between my husband and me. They so get it. I'm terrified that they will hate me and become all messed up in the head, like I am. They will end up making messy decisions like I did out of confused desperation. My parents were so absent in their spirit, and they never seemed to care about what was important to me. I am so ashamed of my weak self. And do you know why? Can I tell you what makes me feel the absolute worst? I am doing the exact same thing to my beautiful children!

I can see my kids withdrawing from me, and it's killing me inside. I try to blame it on adolescence, but I know in my heart that it isn't the whole picture. My little girl who used to talk to me is a stranger now. I feel like she knows what a terrible person I am. How could she not? Yet how could she, really? I have no idea. All I know is that I'm so lost and confused. I've never been more upset.

My husband's so distant and I hate him for it, but the truth is that I have no idea what he thinks about anything, and I wish I knew. My secret dream is that he would just want me again. I want those years back, those years when we were married before the kids . . . even those first few years after my son was born.

I try to talk to my friends, but I'm embarrassed. I have no idea if they'll get it, or talk behind my back. So I down-play most of it. I think about this stuff all the time, I just don't tell anyone. Can I tell you a secret, though? I don't really want to leave him. I just want him to want me. I want him to love me like he used to.

I want to love me. I'm worried that I don't know how.

This dose of brave insight illustrates a raw set of emotions. It reveals how we must translate surface truths into core truths to heal. As this woman boldly lowers her defenses, embraces her role in her own life, and acknowledges previously unspoken fears, she is able to unearth buried feelings. Self-knowledge of this kind removes the brain's need to protect her from the emotional pain by offering her physical pain in its place. Her beach ball can break the surface and drift gently to the corner of the pool. She no longer needs to waste all her resources as she struggles to keep it submerged. Her pain has permission to melt away, and tremendous energy is freed up to experience the full spectrum of her life. This is what happens when the reservoir is lowered. Your body can move into rest-and-repair mode, and no pain, panic attack, or flare-up is required to keep you safe.

Consciousness is the antidote to repression. Continuing to feed denial only perpetuates our brain's natural self-defenses. Beautifully and simply, the practice of JournalSpeak will release you from both denial and pain. Although a person in this position may feel the need to make changes in their life, they need not do so to alleviate their physical symptoms. However, once they've had time to assimilate the new feelings they've become aware of, they will be in a better place to make any changes they choose with calm resolve. I see this process unfold daily in many people's lives, including my own. JournalSpeak leads to personal freedom, and change flows naturally from that.

Your lists are imperative, and at the beginning they can serve as a perfect jumping-off place, but an ongoing JournalSpeak practice is often simply about getting in touch with what is renting the most real estate in your head and heart at the moment. When I find myself wound up and out of touch with my core feelings, I sit for a moment and close my eyes. I ask myself, "What am I feeling most at this very moment?" and whatever arises I just go with it. I write at the top of my journaling page: *Nicole, why are you feeling so angry today?* And then I answer myself. I give myself permission to be real and honest. After all, I'm the only one who's listening. And, mercifully in this case, I'm the only one who needs to hear.

The answer might be "I am angry because I want everyone to leave me alone today, but the kids keep asking for attention. I want to hide. I am angry because I don't want to have self-control and maturity and kindness and compassion for their problems. I want to be selfish and childish too, but I can't. I'm mad at myself because I hold myself to such a high standard as a parent that I feel the need to rise above all of these feelings. I hate that I have to be the grown-up. No one was ever this nice to me! No one ever listened to me the way I listen to them. It's not fair, and I don't want to deal with anything today!"

Keep in mind that strong language can be the vehicle for powerful expression. This doesn't make you a bad person. As my mother always says, "Words have power." So just fucking say the shit you need to say. Remember that the JournalSpeak rant within you is just a little kid screaming to be heard. Take a moment and acknowledge the voice of this small person. It's a five-year-old who is full of unbridled emotions. Their energy has no concern about what's socially appropriate. It is not governed by political correctness. The voice is not polite, not worried about the consequences of what is said. Too often, it's one that's been denied for a lifetime. Oftentimes as children we couldn't speak out for fear of being shamed, or worse. (More on this in Chapter Fifteen when we discuss inner child work.)

These inner youngsters have no interest in being gracious, societally appropriate, or apologizing to anyone for anything. Luckily, you don't need them to. You are a grown-up now, and the people who have created these wounds can't retaliate—not here. You might find yourself feeling any number of ways about your daily life, memories from your past, or frustration around how your personality negotiates challenges and concerns. But feelings aren't facts, and they can't injure you—I promise they hurt less than the chronic pain that has been plaguing you.

YES, EVEN YOU CAN MEDITATE

You've set aside thirty minutes each day for Mindbody work. Twenty minutes are for JournalSpeak. The next ten are for a self-affirming meditation.

This is another point where my clients have balked. They've resisted meditation, protesting that it's "not for them," and, like journaling, it's something that they've tried and dispensed with in the past. So if you just read the phrase *self-affirming meditation* and thought, "Nope!" I recommend hopping back to Chapter Five and reading it again. Resistance is just more TMS—and your skepticism is simply extending this dance with the predators of your repressed emotions. When you find yourself conflicted, look at your resistance with compassion. It has the mentality of a little one who thinks they know best about danger. Thank it kindly for its warning, put it aside, and carry on.

Try "Thanks for sharing. I totally hear you. This is the last thing I feel like doing right now. I also know (from years of Nicole's experience) that this is exactly what is going to make me feel so much better. So guess what? We're doing this now."

So when your JournalSpeak timer goes off at twenty minutes, sit for a ten-minute loving kindness meditation. It can be guided, silent, singing bowls, monks chanting—you name it. The purpose is to hold space for yourself. JournalSpeak may require you to say some extreme things about family, life choices, faith . . . you. It might beckon you to kick, scream, cry, or beg for mercy. This is the kind of raw emotion that is filling the reservoir and presenting a misperceived threat. You need to expel it. Afterward, this can leave you vulnerable and uncertain. Sitting for a consistent self-affirming practice allows you to recenter and remember that you are okay. You may need to say provocative things, but you are saving your own life and sowing the seeds of presence and joy.

Dozens of neuroscience studies have now shown that meditation helps improve mood, quality of sleep, memory, and tension-related symptoms. Many doctors prescribe it to patients who are experiencing heightened anxiety. That's because a regular meditation practice does more than help you focus on the present moment; it actually changes how your nervous system responds to stress. Studies done by researchers at Carnegie Mellon University suggest that these brain changes, coupled with other alterations in your physiology, including your heart rate, improve the ability to regulate your emotions and behaviors. By engaging in these ten minutes of quiet, you can encourage your body to release the repressed emotions ready to break loose—and recalibrate in ways that support calm and focus. You've excavated a lot of hard feelings. The physiological changes that occur in meditation make it easier for you to feel them—and then allow them to go.

There's no one way to take this time for yourself. You can download an app to walk you through a guided meditation. You can chant your favorite mantra or count your breaths. You can even put on some soothing music and just *be*. It really doesn't matter. Just do whatever will help you to be still, and send love to that sweet, scared little kid that lives within you. They're trying their very best. They aren't sure yet if things will be okay. They need reassurance from the grown you, the one who is stepping into their power and has the ability to reparent that small, wobbly one.

Look, if I can meditate, anyone can meditate. I am, by nature, a fast-talking, fast-moving, anxious, and frenetic soul. Establishing a daily practice wasn't easy, but I took it on with the same mindset as I do JournalSpeak: This is self-care and it will make me feel better in so many ways, so I'm going to stop whining and just do it. Little by slowly it revealed its value in the changes I saw in myself. Body as proof, once again! I became more grounded, less nervous, more able to slow down. Meditation is not only scientifically proven to rewire neural pathways for equanimity, but in the context of JournalSpeak, it proves to be a safe haven of personal forgiveness after the stuff you need to say.

NOW, THROW IT AWAY

Once you have finished your JournalSpeak and meditation, it's time to unburden yourself. You've been brave enough to show up to the page with honesty, and you've done your best to release any attendant shame via meditation. But there's still one more step.

Whatever you wrote during your twenty minutes, it's time to throw those words away. If you journaled into a notebook or diary, tear out the pages, rip them up, and throw them into a garbage can where no one could possibly see. If you have a shredder, go nuts. I've had clients who burned the pages in their fireplaces or in a can in the backyard. If you used a laptop, perhaps composing an email with no recipient or creating an untitled document, delete the draft. The whole point is to cleanse yourself of those negative feelings. You don't need to carry them anymore. As one client mentioned during my years of private practice, "It's like blowing your nose into a tissue! Throw it away. You don't need to look at it again."

The reasons for disposing of your JournalSpeak are twofold. First, once the feelings arise, the job has been done. The waters of your reservoir will begin to recede. Second, JournalSpeak is a language that could easily be misinterpreted by loved ones, friends, or employers. Protect yourself by not leaving your journal around for others to discover. In the case that you want to keep your writing for other therapeutic purposes (such as sharing with a trusted therapist or friend, which can sometimes be helpful), just be mindful of keeping it private. You are participating in this exercise to free yourself of chronic pain, anxiety, and the symptoms that have plagued you for years. You must feel safe for it to work.

As you set forth on this voyage, let me leave you with a piece I've titled "The MindScience of JournalSpeak." Allow it to be a script that you carry in your pocket—a conversation between yourself and you. Let it serve as a gentle reminder of all that we've discussed thus far and launch you into this transformative practice with peace and resolve.

THE MINDSCIENCE OF JOURNALSPEAK

If the purpose of my pain is to deter me from thinking my unthinkable things, then simply allowing myself to think the unthinkable things disables this natural protective mechanism. In this process, however, something happens which is very natural. I begin to consider that thinking these things will "hurt me worse." This is part of the science. The brain, in its estimation, wants me to avoid focusing on them to shield me from their "dangerous" qualities. The problem is that if I stop there and cease to think about the things, then my brain's last vestige of protective mechanism wins, and the feelings are repressed once again. Then, pain and more pain. The cycle can't do anything but continue.

But if I show up every day, like a warrior, and think of them again, and write them again, and sit with them again, I am training my primitive brain to understand that I am safe. I am evolving right here in my own space and time. I am showing my nervous system, over and over, that I don't need this pain or crippling chronic anxiety to protect me from my feelings. I can sit with my big emotions, be brave, and feel whatever is necessary to convince my brain that I don't need protection.

The thoughts that lead me away from my JournalSpeak can feel so logical. This is also part of the science. The brain is cunning and crafty. It uses my voice. These are "my" thoughts. They say, "You should be embarrassed you're still worrying about these things." They say, "You will launch yourself right into negativity and symptoms if you think about this again." These messages sound right to me be-cause my brain prioritizes my survival. It is trying to guide me into a "safe" space. But this space is only safe in the unsafest way. It is one of obsessing about my symptoms and my failure to get rid of them, or perhaps planning an-other doctor's visit to make sure I'm okay. My brain is try-ing to help me survive in the best way it knows how—it is, it believes, keeping me alive.

My whole system needs a renovation. It is operating with primitive tools. It doesn't realize that I can feel these things a million times. I am strong, and I can do it. It is my responsibility to teach it this because my brain is in control of my body and the way it feels. My brain is completely and utterly the ruler of my experiences and sensations. I may not have immediate control of its natural reaction to stimuli, whether emotional or otherwise. I do, however, have control of my intentional mind. And my mind is infinite and powerful. My mind knows that my brain loves me, but it needs training. If I value feeling good and at peace, it is my job to retrain my brain to react properly to the proper stimuli.

For example, if there is a predator chasing me, then my primitive system is right on. The stimulus of being chased and having my life in literal danger is the correct one to launch me into fight or flight. Go, nervous system! Nice work. Thank you for making me run a little faster, and think a little quicker, and respond with laser focus. Thank you because I am alive, and perhaps without your immediate assistance I would be dead.

There are places, however, where you need a little updating. I don't need you to react with that fight-or-flight response to the rising awareness of my feelings. You don't need to protect me because I am scared about my decisions. I am not in danger when I worry about being judged by others, or when my personal relationships are not what I'd hoped for. I can handle (however uncomfortably) my children's uncertain happiness, the way my parents treated me as a child, and the patterns I've developed as a result. It is my job to show you the difference between real and perceived danger. I do this by telling you, over and over, what I really feel. Little by slowly you will realize that I need not run away from these thoughts, or freeze in the high grass so they might not notice me, or fight them with the power of a hundred soldiers.

You will realize, by and by, that I am thinking these thoughts and having these feelings and I am not in peril. They are just thoughts and feelings. I am still here. Nothing has swallowed me whole because I regret my decisions, or I haven't spoken up for myself, or I lied about something, or I've gotten myself in over my head. It might not feel good, but it's not going to injure me, so you can stop protecting me by giving me something "real" to focus on.

I know just telling you once isn't enough. I need to tell you every day, again and again, by sharing with you my dirty, ugly, unpleasant, shameful, embarrassing, terrifying, devastating, enraging thoughts: my JournalSpeak. *By doing this, I prove to you by feeling them and knowing them that I won't die. You will learn eventually and stop sending signals, telling my body that I need pain to distract and protect me.*

When I tell myself my truth over and over, it will fail to hold the power it once held. As I do, I accept that when one thing loses its charge, another seemingly new one will take its place with a similar charge. And then I will think, speak, and write about that one. I need only communicate to myself, but I must communicate. I cannot stand quietly by, because if I do, my primitive system will take the baton and protect me however it sees fit. This is no longer acceptable to me. I choose to feel my ugly, uncomfortable, unpleasant feelings rather than live in pain.

As I adopt this way of living, emotions will cease to frighten me, because I'll know that life is just like that—every day I might think and feel upsetting things, but they will not kill me. I am safe. My life will be my own. My pain will flow through me as it must, but it will not own me. I will live a life of truth and choice. I will evolve to the greatest version of myself, and I will be free.

This is the way forward. You are brave enough and strong enough to take it. After all, look at all you've withstood so far.

●

Michael's Recovery from Back Pain, Sciatica, and Three Back Surgeries—Age 25 (Western United States)

My name is Michael Porter Jr. and I play on the Denver Nuggets. People know me as MPJ. I've been in the NBA for six years now, and I've been playing basketball since I was three years old. My back problems started when I was a sophomore in high school. I fell on my back during a layup, and at the time I thought I just didn't give myself enough time to recover because it continually got more and more sore. At that point, the pain was localized in my lower back, and it got increasingly severe throughout high school. My junior year rolled around, and then my senior year. The pain continued to get worse. I played through it, determined not to let it stop me from achieving my dreams.

I ended up at the University of Missouri as the number one recruit in the country. I was supposed to be the number one pick in the NBA draft the following year, but my back problems kept interfering. I went to see all types of chiropractors and physical therapists, to no avail. It seemed that every time I saw someone new, my back problems became more severe.

A few months down the line and the pain was now in two places and the sciatica was debilitating. I saw a doctor who said that I had a protruding herniated disc, and I would need surgery. I was consumed with worry and fear for my future. I had no idea what "degenerative disc disease" was, but it sounded bad. I now know it's a natural part of aging, and even just growing for a guy like me who's almost seven feet tall. Looking back, I can see how that phrase triggered real terror in my brain. I recall one chiropractor saying, "Man, if you don't get this fixed with surgery, you're never going to play in the NBA."

So I got the surgery in college and sat out for three or four months. I felt better initially, but four months later the pain was worse than ever. I went back to the doctors. They said that the disc disease had moved up a level. I was devastated. The draft occurred, and I dropped to fourteenth. It was crushing. I underwent another surgery, and another: three back surgeries total—L4/L5, L3/L4, and L2/L3. Nothing relieved my pain for long.

I was still playing in the NBA by the grace of God, but I would have flare-ups every month or two. When they were major, I wasn't able to work out for two to three days. This just isn't sustainable for someone who has to play at my level. I was constantly anxious about when the next one would come.

In the summer of 2023, I was staying in L.A. when my back flared badly. I got to thinking, "Man, there's got to be something out there that can help me!" And then I remembered Dr. Sarno. I had read *Healing Back Pain* and it resonated with me. But at the time I wasn't ready to put my full trust in the idea that I didn't need more surgery. Now I found myself curious. One night, I came across Nicole Sachs's four-part series called *Healing Yourself*. A lightbulb went off. I understood that if I wanted to get better, I needed to put in the time and do the work.

I know many people don't get the chance to speak directly to Nicole, so I am blessed to say that I was able to get her counsel. She told me her story and heard mine, and she explained exactly how I could get better. I started applying her methods, consistently, every day. I was not messing around. I was JournalSpeaking twenty minutes a day, meditating, and truly believing that my back problems were the result of the mind/body connection. I learned all about the brain science, self-compassion, and inner child work. You might think a guy like me would dismiss all this touchy-feely stuff, but I was really giving it a chance. I wanted my life. I wanted my career and my greatest joy, playing basketball.

As I write this, I'm about to play my twenty-fourth game of the season. I haven't even come close to missing a game because of back pain. I'm consistently getting the second-highest minutes of play on the team. If I ever ache at all, it's just the occasional soreness that anyone would get. I've missed so many games because of my back. This year, I'm looking forward to playing in the most games I've played in a season since turning pro. A friend told me the other day that I'm playing like the kid he remembers from high school, maybe the best basketball of my life.

This process has changed my perspective on pain. It's changed my perspective on life and how we need to deal with our emotions. The body does not operate all alone as muscles, organs, and nerves; it's physical, emotional, mental, and spiritual. You can't just pay attention to the physical and expect yourself to be thriving and healthy. Being human is multifaceted.

The biggest gift that this healing journey has given me is the understanding that pain is part of becoming whole as a person. You get to know yourself. And you learn to have self-compassion because your JournalSpeak connects the dots of your life experiences. You can move forward in a loving and caring way.

CHAPTER 9

EVOLVE YOUR JOURNALSPEAK

S o here we are. You are living the dream, doing the work. A big question I get as people travel along this path is "What happens if on any given day my lists don't feel relevant or pressing?" Or "How do I keep going deeper once I've exhausted them?" Or "What is the most effective way to continue moving forward?" Yes, yes. These are great questions. Let's answer them together.

Recall that we are so "frightened" by our big feelings that we *reflexively* repress them. As you know by now, this begins out of survival—these big feelings make us feel unsafe. Over the years you've collected emotional reactions, and since you are ill-equipped to process them, they get dumped into your imagined reservoir. Of course, no one could possibly process the amount of emotive input a person receives on a daily basis. It's not just the struggle of being alive with all of your current responsibilities and pressures. It's every trigger that brings you unconsciously back to a childhood wound. It's your very personality that creates the lens through which every experience is filtered.

Once you've begun your excavation, fear and resistance can cause you to question and doubt even more effectively. Maybe the symptom imperative has kicked in, and you've found yourself reunited with Dr. Google at three a.m., searching for the next medical fix. You are not alone. Let's talk about your reservoir. It's really the culprit here.

Let's review the core concepts. The reservoir keeps reaching maximum density—that's okay. It's just part of being human. When it threatens to spill over and inform your conscious mind that you are filled to the brim with rage, fear, grief, despair, or shame, a symptom pops up. This is because in this overflowing state, your conscious brain begins to become aware of how stuck and hopeless you feel over the things you cannot control. Although these feelings are manageable and safe when given the right form of expression and support, an overflowing reservoir sends danger signals equivalent to a survival risk to the brain and nervous system. "You cannot feel this stuff! If you know how much you resent your kids, you might drive away and never come back! If you feel the conflicts in your relationship, you may want to leave it! If you know how you really see yourself, the inner loathing could eat you alive!"

So, as you know, the nervous system zooms into fight or flight and sends protection in the form of pain. Remember that pain, in its essence, *is* protective. When we cut ourselves, it hurts so we are sure to clean it and keep it from getting infected. An infection, unmitigated, is a survival risk. Chronic pain is serving the same purpose, however unwelcome.

Just keep reminding your brain: the crazy (and incredible) thing is that these feelings are not dangerous at all. They are normal and human. Every single person feels them. When you have the freedom and awareness to acknowledge their existence, you can deal with them. The moment you are able to pause and replace your fear with curiosity, you can turn toward them. Evolving your JournalSpeak practice involves dipping a ladle into the reservoir and dumping it out. The moment it is no longer at the edge of spilling over, the pain signals are no longer necessary. Your nervous system, which has been acting as a sentinel to protect you, can stand down. It receives the message: There is nothing dangerous here. Let's remind ourselves of the key topics that commonly spark questions and struggles as you JournalSpeak your way out of pain.

CONSISTENCY

It takes time to become proficient in JournalSpeak. Each one of us has an inner child—one whose voice was too often ignored in times of struggle. Our wellness is tied directly to letting them speak. Your JournalSpeak will not look like mine or anyone else's. You will find the language you need to let your core feelings rise. We begin the Mindbody work with Dr. Sarno's original Childhood (or Past Stressors), Daily Life, and Personality chart, but it does not end there. Life is not static. Although you start by examining the feelings you've been repressing over time, you continue by saying what you need to say to keep your reservoir from getting too full.

This practice is more than doable if you're willing to embrace the dreaded C word: *consistency*. Anything feels easy to do once or twice, like working out, eating healthily, or taking a yoga class. But we all know that the only practices that yield enduring results are those we do with regularity. If you want to retrain your brain to stop protecting you with pain, anxiety, symptoms, and conditions, you need to dip a ladle into this reservoir and pour it out *on the regular.*

Although your symptoms are not a life sentence by any means, until they decline considerably, I am going to ask you to do your JournalSpeak practice every day. As we discussed in Chapter Six, consistency is key when it comes to disarming this natural and protective reflex. When we are in sustained fight or flight and the reservoir is at maximum density, inflammation, muscle constriction and spasm, nerve zings, and other unpleasant bodily reactions are on a hair trigger. Doing the work to lower it is key to bringing you into rest and repair—and, consequently, rewiring your brain for wellness.

RESISTANCE

Consistent work can be triggering, because it calls out all the fears that might have been lurking in the shadows. I know it sounds nuts, but it can be "scary" to be out of pain. You might ask yourself: *What if I am no longer comfortable asking for help? What if people don't pay attention to me anymore? What if I'm not as loved as I thought I was?* Maybe you believe, deep down, that you aren't worthy of a pain-free and fulfilling life. Perhaps you're worried that being free of chronic issues just isn't in the cards. All these fears might be blaring in the background, telling your conscious mind:

An emotional exercise could never cure a physical problem.

This is too good to be true.

My doctor told me I have this condition.

My mother had the same thing.

My MRI says so.

I'm allergic to food.

I'm sensitive to chemicals.

I'm predisposed.

There's evidence in my X-ray.

I've had this since I was a kid.

This is just who I am.

I hear you, and I get it. But that is just another face of resistance, and as you continue to show up to the page, it will wane.

WHY TWENTY MINUTES?

Many of my clients over the years have gotten stuck on the idea of twenty minutes. "Why twenty? Why not thirty? What about ten? Might five minutes be enough?" Let's discuss.

During my first appointment with Dr. Sarno, he recommended that I journal about my feelings for thirty minutes in the morning and thirty minutes in the evening. I remember wanting to ask him, "I mentioned I have two toddlers, right?" Although I knew it would be a challenge, I earnestly tried to follow his prescription for weeks. I knew I needed to do so to stop my nervous system from protecting me with such vehemence.

After a while, I realized that I didn't need to set aside an hour every day. As I honed my practice, I noticed that I could get to the heart of my core feelings in about twenty minutes. I paid attention to my clients and the feedback I was getting from my online community, and twenty minutes continued to be the sweet spot—it's enough time to do the work you need to do to lower your emotional reservoir. It's also manageable, no matter how busy or tired you are. Trust me: If I can find thirty minutes in my day for my Journal-Speak/meditation practice, you can, too.

Still, that said, some of you might find that you are hitting a rather formidable resistance barrier as you try to fill twenty minutes. Recently, a woman trying JournalSpeak told me, "I wrote for eight minutes, but then I couldn't think of what else to say."

This is a place where you need to push past your nervous system's protective stance of resistance, exhaustion, and excuses. Ask yourself, *Is what I'm writing real and true?* If not, dig deeper—find the words that convey those feelings about the subject matter. Sometimes I actually stop midsentence if my JournalSpeak is not feeling authentic, and write *Nicole, what is real and true?* and then I continue, *What is real and true is* _____. Completing this sentence often gets me to the heart of the resistance I might be facing.

What is real and true is that I'm tired and I can't stand thinking about this stuff anymore.

What is real and true is that I don't want to do this; I'd rather take a pill.

What is real and true is that I'm fucking pissed I have to do this work in the first place.

And so on . . .

Another JournalSpeak hack is to pick up your pen or your keyboard and document your inner child's rantings:

This is so stupid. I have nothing to write about. I don't know what I'm doing and have no idea how getting a hand cramp is going to help my knee pain. How come everyone else but me can manage twenty minutes? What is wrong with me?

These tactics will often kick your JournalSpeak session back into high gear. Just keep reminding yourself:

I am saving my own life. I am rewiring my neural pathways for optimal health and wellness. I am giving myself a gift of which I can't possibly yet know the value. This is power, and it is mine.

Before you know it, your words—your voice—will take you where you need to go. Keep your pen or your fingers moving. The discomfort of having to push through your resistance is breeding ground for epiphany. Like anything else, your barriers will dissolve if you can sit with your traumatic memories and complex feelings and let them have their say.

LIFE CAN BE LIFEY

Let's be frank—life is lifey sometimes. Although it's not ideal, there will be days that finding twenty minutes is simply not possible. Something comes up that throws your carefully planned schedule out the window. The kids won't respect your boundaries. Your boss shortens your lunch hour so you can help finish up a big project. Shit happens, and we all have to adapt.

On days like these, I recommend doing what you can with what you have. If you only have five minutes, take that time to bullet out what's bothering you. I've had clients sit in the park during their lunch break, sandwich in hand, and write out their core feelings on a napkin. You can make some space, even on the busiest of days, to ladle out your emotional reservoir. Especially in stressful, unpredictable times, it is essential to do what you can to ensure it doesn't overflow.

EVOLVING YOUR PRACTICE

After you've been JournalSpeaking for a while, you may notice that your original Childhood (or Past Stressors), Daily Life, and Personality lists have been X-ed out like a winning bingo card. You've addressed many longstanding issues—and you are beginning to feel the results in your body. *Thanksgiving 1996* doesn't have the same hold on you now that you've acknowledged some of your unresolved feelings around it. You've taken the time to examine the daily, common struggles of your life, and you've given your principal personality traits their day in the sun.

This is not to say that you shouldn't revisit any of these bullets as many times as you need. There is great value in returning to something until it fails to hold the charge it once held. Your lists are meant to be a jumping-off point—a way to start writing about your feelings to help you understand their connection to your pain. But JournalSpeak is not a "one [or even fifty] and done" kind of thing. Some items may need more than one session. Others—the real biggies that still hold sway over your life—may need regular excavation. Please, never shame yourself for this. You are not more damaged than the next guy because you have to talk about your mother *again*. Each JournalSpeak journey is unique, as each of us is.

Because we are living, breathing creatures who interact with the outside world every single day, new and related issues will always come up. This is to be expected and welcomed, mostly because we have no other choice! When you find that the items on your lists aren't demanding your attention any longer, the work doesn't stop. It's just time to identify the issues that may be threatening to overflow your emotional reservoir in the *right now*. As you pass through this new world of self-excavation and reflection, it's helpful to have a little guidance on giving the present moment the attention it deserves. This is time well spent—to sit for just a moment longer with ways in which you can stay curious in your practice.

When people reach out to me and tell me they don't think they have anything more to write about, I assure them, "Oh, honey, not to fear. There's plenty more to find." Fortunately or unfortunately, this being human is not over till the human part of it is over. There is always more. From my heart, I find this "endlessness" to be a positive thing. As I evolve my own practice, as I am a work in progress just like you, I often sit with wonder and gratitude for the lessons that continue to be revealed. I am here to grow. I am here to live and love with passion and veracity. This is only possible when I stay forever inquisitive about what is lurking in the places I might be enticed to avoid.

In the end, feeling like we've "seen it all" is just another form of resistance. Luckily, there are strategies to help you overcome your blockages. You can go beyond the lists to detect what, in your life, in this moment, requires the voice of JournalSpeak.

One way to keep things moving is to revise your lists. As you work through different items, it may be time for a redo. Put your old inventory aside and once again create a table with three headings: Childhood (or Past Stressors), Daily Life, and Personality. Take a moment, breathe, and consider what items should be on them right now. They may differ from the ones you added when you started JournalSpeaking. They may even be different from the elements that seemed most important *yesterday.*

You are growing and changing, and this is the work of a lifetime. This doesn't mean it's a *life sentence.* I don't JournalSpeak every day anymore. But it is a tool that will never forsake me, and I use it when I need to. Your JournalSpeak journey is just that—yours—and you get to determine what experiences, issues, or core feelings require excavation. I'll only caution you not to revise your lists to avoid a specific item. You know what I'm talking about.

There may be a notation that you've specifically sidestepped because you are afraid to talk about it—or worry about what kind of feelings it might unleash. *If that's where you are right now, go right to that biggie.* Start writing about that topic during your next JournalSpeak session. The very fact that you continue to avoid it is telling you it's time.

Another tactic is to ask yourself the following question as you begin a session: What is occupying the most space ("renting the most real estate," as you'll hear me say) in my head *right now*? What feeling may be manifesting itself as irritation or annoyance—or, worse, the beginnings of a migraine or a twinge in your "bad shoulder"? Figure out what is taking up all the space on your bench, and start writing about it. You never know where your Journal-Speak might take you. The thought you begin with is just a bunny in the fresh snow—place it down and let it run, back and forth, over and around. You might start at the soccer game with the obnoxious screaming parent in front of you and find yourself in your childhood bedroom listening to your parents fight. It's a beautiful thing to replace your fear with curiosity and go for the ride with the sweet little one inside who is so grateful for your attention after being alone for so long.

On days when I'm not sure where to start, I like to take a mini inventory. As I sit down to do my JournalSpeak, I bang out five things in recent history that really angered me, scared me, saddened me, shamed me, or made me anxious. Maybe they are simply things I can't stop thinking about. They don't have to be related, and they don't have to be "big." They just have to have left an impression. Once I've noted these antagonists, I pick one to write about. Maybe it's the one that's most egregious, something that really pushed my boundaries. Perhaps it's an incident that's got me ruminating—I know I'm creating a "tape" of it in my head as I'm trying to get through my day. Or maybe, just maybe, there's an item that my mind recoils at discussing. As I said before, if you have that visceral reaction to it, that should be your prompt. It is for me, on such a day. Just start writing.

Paying attention to your current feelings is a vital way to evolve your practice—and make sure that today's problems don't become tomorrow's reservoir fillers.

USE A LITERAL PROMPT

When you've spent the majority of your life unconsciously repressing, it's not always second nature to let things surface. Sometimes it's good to have a prompt to get you going. One that I love personally is Tara Brach's timeless question, "What am I unwilling to feel?" Some others I often suggest to clients include:

_____ *really makes my blood boil.*

I wish I had said _____ *to so-and-so when she confronted me.*

I feel so _____ *about that recent decision.*

I wish I could change _____ *about my (kids, partner, friend, brother, job).*

I still believe I have to _____ *to be loved and accepted.*

I'm afraid to admit this, even to myself, but

_____.

My biggest secret is _____.

I hate _____ about myself.

I avoid feeling _____ at all costs.

I wish I were brave enough to say _____ to my mom (dad, sister, partner, friend).

I'm scared of _____ the most.

What's really making me hopeless right now is _____ if I'm being totally honest.

I refuse to accept the fact that _____.

I feel so much shame about _____ even though it's been years.

I am enraged by the way _____ behaves.

I feel like _____ is missing from my life.

I am afraid to grieve (confront, accept, express) _____.

Find your electronic copy of these prompts at www.nicolesachs.com/prompts.

Pick a prompt that calls to you. Then the same rules apply. Start writing and keep your pen (fingers) moving for twenty minutes. You never know what you might discover. Don't forget about the ten minutes of self-affirming meditation when you're done. This is painful stuff, and rightfully so. Your brain would not send in an army of protection against feelings that did not hold a potent charge.

You know what's at stake here. Your life is too important to remain in the state you're in. When you can unveil your fears, your rage, your shame, your despair, your grief, and other powerhouse emotions, you'll be opened to possibilities you'd never imagined. It creates space. You'll begin to picture the life you want—the relationships you wish to cultivate. You'll start to know that you can make things happen for yourself. This is what inspiration feels like.

With consistent work, you will see your pain begin to recede. The results may not be immediate, but they will come. As you become more proficient in allowing your inner child to speak freely (much more on this in Chapter Thirteen) and inviting those ugly and inappropriate sentiments to rise, rest and repair will become a consistent state of being. The difference you feel will astonish you—body, mind, and spirit. Be bravely regular with your practice, and watch the cracks of light grow and deepen. Freedom awaits.

•

Lauren's Recovery from Chronic Migraines, Anxiety, and Panic Attacks—Age 35 (Northeastern United States)

I started getting migraines in college, but as-needed medications got rid of them, and I lived a full life. However, once I got into graduate school to become a physical therapist, the migraines started becoming severe and more frequent. I began a slew of prescriptions. I also developed severe anxiety. Like "terrified my husband was going to die every time he left the house" anxiety. I saw a physician and was diagnosed with generalized anxiety disorder (GAD) and was given more meds. Somehow I made it through school, graduated with my doctorate, and began working.

Shortly after I had my first child, everything broke. I was hospitalized a few times a month because of the severity of the migraines. They lasted for weeks without any reprieve. I had to get dihydroergotamine (DHE) infusions, which would make me sick, but they were the only thing to break the cycle.

My neurologist strongly recommended I stop working to focus on getting better. We sold our home, downsized, and I went on disability. We didn't want to stop living life, and we'd always planned on having a second child. After much deliberation, we decided to get pregnant again. We didn't want to live with the regret of not trying.

Shortly after having my son, however, I was hospitalized because my vitals were irregular and I was constantly dizzy. Through that hospitalization and subsequent follow-up visits I was diagnosed with postural orthostatic tachycardia syndrome (POTS). My resting heart rate was in the nineties. *Resting!* That means that just getting up and walking around would cause it to soar as high as 180. I couldn't shower because the symptoms were so bad. My husband literally washed my hair in the sink as if I were at a salon. But this was no spa day! I spent about twenty-five to twenty-seven days a month with a migraine. I was a stay-at-home mom who sent her kids to daycare. I was miserable. I started having panic attacks. I couldn't manage living.

One weekend when I just couldn't take it anymore, I asked my family if I could go away alone to a cabin. This was my rock bottom. Then, through what I fully believe was divine intervention, I came across Nicole's work online. I binged countless hours of her podcast over the next three days learning about the Mindbody connection and chronic pain.

As soon as I understood the concepts, belief was no problem for me. I was a poster child for TMS. I had plenty of childhood trauma— each parent getting divorced and remarrying three times. My dad was in the military, so we moved more times than I can count. I remember feeling unsafe on so many occasions. Plus, when I was eighteen and finally ready to move away and start a new life, I was diagnosed with an extremely rare cancer that altered my life forever.

Knowledge alone of the Mindbody connection reduced my migraines by half; I was averaging only seventeen a month. *Only!* But to me it meant a return to life. At that time, I was not ready to really dive in and do the work. As Nicole says, "True readiness is everything." When my migraines hit hard again after having baby number three, I decided to hit the healing hard back.

I started JournalSpeak. Making the lists about childhood, current stressors, and personality traits opened my eyes to how much crap was under the surface. I had some digging to do! Thankfully, I had the first part down—belief. And once I accepted that I had to do it, the next part—the work—came surprisingly naturally to me. Sometimes you just have to decide that you are going to do a hard thing, no matter what. I was amazed at how powerful writing for twenty minutes could be! I would start on one topic and end up twenty minutes later in a completely different rabbit hole. So many emotions were felt and released during this time. Some things, like my cancer diagnosis as a teenager, I had to hash out over days and weeks. But I was healing myself, and it was powerful. I learned so much about who I am that I swear it was worth it even if my actual symptoms never changed.

The physical healing did come. I noticed I kept getting alerts from my iWatch that my resting heart rate was lower. Then lower. It dropped into the sixties, a healthy level. I had exercise tolerance again. I rode my bike five days a week. The POTS was gone. The migraines were no longer chronic.

I was changing my body in real time. Month after month, the headaches became less frequent, and their severity drastically reduced. I learned to not fear the pain but instead ask what it was trying to tell me. I partnered with it. I embraced it—something I thought I could never do. I'd always said I needed a new head because this one was against me. But it was actually my mindset and awareness that needed to shift!

This brings me to the third part of the work—self-compassion. This is what came last to me, as I didn't realize how unkind I had been to myself my whole life. I used Kristin Neff's offerings to dive into this part of my healing. I would have laughed myself out of the room a couple years ago if you said I was going to meditate. I thought that I was just not the type that could sit quietly. My personality was too uptight and controlling. I simply could not relax.

No longer.

This transformation has been nothing short of magical. I am so different now, and yet the same. I can recognize that I am who I've always been, but I needed some real education on how to know myself. The pain was an important part of my life story. There was nothing wrong or broken with me that needed to be fixed. In the end, the whole experience was simply a moment of suffering for me. Without it, I would not have found the healing and growth I sorely needed.

I've become the person who is "grateful for my pain"—something I never thought possible. I have gotten off all medications for anxiety and migraines. I live free of chronic conditions. It is astounding, it is amazing, and it is my life.

CHAPTER 10

FINDING THE ANSR AND LETTING YOUR BODY BE YOUR PROOF

A s you may have already begun to personally experience (and can see in the stories of people who've walked this path), the proper Mindbody mindset paired with a JournalSpeak practice has remarkable power to lower your emotional reservoir and allow the body to settle into a restorative state—without the need for pain or chronic symptoms. As you build JournalSpeak into your daily routine, you'll be able not only to release past sufferings but to stop your mind from tamping down the core feelings that come with newer situations.

It takes time and patience, but you will witness firsthand new insights into how your nervous system responds to your environment. Human beings, by nature, are reactive creatures. When you are not self-aware enough to understand the aspects of your world—your family, your work, your insecurities—that cause you to repress emotions, the body must register and express the overflow. Instead of (ideally) meeting every challenge with calm consideration, you have no choice but to constantly recoil from your triggers much like you do when you pull your hand off a hot stove.

In the world of stored trauma and unresolved feelings, these responses have been survival techniques. You are finally ready to evolve away from them.

There comes a time when you become experienced enough with JournalSpeak to understand that you're living in the ANSR. As a society, we are so good at delineating the problem, yet we struggle against the current to find accessible solutions. As I've developed this work over years of practice, I've come to find myself calmly and confidently in a perpetual "flow state" when it comes to my health. This is what I offer you in these pages: a way to embrace a whole new way of living. Let's take a step back and consider each of your emotional experiences in four parts: Allow, Name, Stay, Release.

Fun fact: I was recording a podcast episode, live, the moment I realized that the acronym of this process sounded like "the answer" (ANSR). I was obviously very delighted with myself. So, the ANSR it became!

Doing this work is a treasure hunt—we must acknowledge a lifetime of experiences, some very painful, shaming, upsetting, and confusing. You, as a soft, chewy human, are naturally resistant to allowing these experiences to be seen, felt, and acknowledged. As we've discussed, this is not just cognizant human defiance. Your resistance comes from the unconscious processes operating under the cover of darkness in your brain. As we open ourselves to the transformations possible within this practice, we begin to learn how to manage any new, complicated feelings that may arise.

We embrace living within the ANSR.

ANSR is the framework within which we can view both old and new core feelings with the kind of awareness that allows us to process them and let them go. There are new challenges ahead—there always are—and the ANSR provides an effectual path so you never have to worry about your reservoir overflowing again.

Here are the definitions of each aspect of the ANSR framework:

Allow—*Consider that since emotions are the "predator" from which the nervous system and brain are protecting us, we must* allow *each moment, story, relationship, experience, et cetera and the attendant emotions to rise and be present. This is not meant to be overwhelming and should not cause undue anxiety. Nothing will flood you all at once. Allowing is simply an awareness that if healing requires knowing these things, you must allow them to surface and recognize their power.*

Name—*Once you have allowed a memory, trigger, or story to surface, it's time to* name *it for what it is. Naming is JournalSpeak. It is synonymous with "doing the work." It is a process that takes our past experiences, traumatic memories, and responses to daily life and tasks us with writing out all of our associated feelings. JournalSpeak is invaluable in effective naming because human beings think at lightning speed. When we slow down to write, we are able to view things in a new and evolving light. This makes space for epiphany. Slowness invites the brain to understand and accept that there is no danger in feeling these uncomfortable, yet not unsafe, emotions. I know I'm repeating myself, but it's important to say it again: Uncomfortable does not equal unsafe. And thank goodness for that, because the road to different is uncomfortable.*

Stay—*All animals, including human beings, are wired to run from danger. It takes mindful intention and consciousness to* stay. *Staying, in this process, means resisting the urge to escape. Intentionally staying with your feelings once they are* *named sends a message of safety to the nervous system. Your natural impulse may be to flee from what you uncover in your JournalSpeak practice. It is an act of love for oneself and the inner child to stay and to be the parent that perhaps you never had.*

Release—*Letting go of the grip that your hurtful life's experiences have on you is the natural result of allowing, naming, and staying. People ask me all the time, "How do I release my pain and suffering? How do I discharge this anguish? It has such a hold on me!" And I remind you with love and empathy that* release *cannot be forced, pushed, or begged for. The nervous system perceives your desire to be different (than you are) as fear. Desperation for release creates more inflammation and constriction in your systems and dumps more content into the reservoir. Release will come organically as you work through allowing, naming, and staying.*

Put them all together and you have a framework that will ultimately allow you to leave your chronic pain and anxiety behind—and move into a space of authenticity that doesn't feel threatening.

As you read these definitions, you may be thinking, "That's great—but *how*, exactly, do I incorporate the ANSR into my Mindbody work? How can I harness its power to help me heal?"

I'm glad you asked. As you become more accustomed to JournalSpeak, you can use this framework to guide you as you write. Eventually, even outside your daily JournalSpeak practice, you can leverage the ANSR to help you cope with any life situation. Let's dive into each aspect.

ALLOW

You begin this healing process by opening the door—by allowing your life and personality to be seen. Remember, you are the only one who needs to appreciate what is revealed. This fact provides much-needed salve at the beginning—you don't need to confront anyone or change your circumstances to be free of chronic suffering. In moments of hesitation, remind yourself that you have agency. You can act with intention. You can decide to stop doing what you've always done, because the resulting pain, symptoms, and general discomfort are no longer serving you. As you become aware of what you need to examine by making your lists and considering your triggers and traumatic memories, allow the feelings and experiences to enter. Invite them in like Rumi's poem "The Guest House."

"The Guest House"

BY RUMI

This being human is a guest house.
Every morning a new arrival.
A joy, a depression, a meanness,
some momentary awareness comes
as an unexpected visitor.
Welcome and entertain them all!
Even if they're a crowd of sorrows,
who violently sweep your house
empty of its furniture,
still, treat each guest honorably.
He may be clearing you out
for some new delight.
The dark thought, the shame, the malice,

meet them at the door laughing,
and invite them in.
Be grateful for whomever comes,
because each has been sent
as a guide from beyond.

I often tell people that allowing is like being on the kindergarten carpet. You are sitting with all your "little shmoos," as Ram Dass calls them. They are your neuroses, your hurt feelings, your resentments, and your upsetting memories (as best you can recall on any given day). They are flawed and imperfect, as are everyone's. As you calmly sit on the colorful carpet with them, another one may knock at the door. You might remember a time when something gutted you or find yourself triggered by what happened earlier that day. All of a sudden, you are right back with those feelings of rage that were so potent in middle school. This is good stuff! Don't resist these visitors. Whatever comes up, it's okay.

Everyone is welcome here. Scoot over on the carpet and make room for each little shmoo to sit. The carpet is infinite, so there is nothing to worry about. As long as you're willing to look up and make room, you are moving in the direction of wellness. You just have to stop fighting so hard to block these emotions out! That's what we're doing together when we allow. We are making room. We are holding space. We are practicing equanimity and beginning to realize that being with these (sometimes ugly-looking) parts of ourselves is tolerable and safe.

As you do this, you challenge the natural barriers that arise with allowing: negative self-talk encouraging you to give up, exhaustion that the nervous system sends as protection, and numbness that accompanies overwhelming feelings. Acknowledge the resistance, but keep the door open.

NAME

Naming is where JournalSpeak comes in. It allows the nervous system to give up its reflexive protective stance. You will come to see that pain signals fire only when you are "in danger."

As my colleague and Oxford-trained biologist Gigi Cockell teaches, it helps to think of your symptoms like a red, cylindrical fire alarm, the glaring lights spinning round and round within the chamber. Every day, when you give your symptoms your full attention, carrying them with you to doctor's appointments, treatments, and procedures, you are, in effect, dousing the alarm with a fire hose again and again. Take a step back and think about this effort you're making. Then consider the results of that effort. The truth is, no matter how soaked the alarm gets, it will never stop screaming. Why? (You know why.) Because the problem is not actually the alarm. The alarm is just *communicating to you* that there is a problem.

The real concern is the fire.

In this case, the fire is your repressed emotional world and stored trauma. It is raging inside, bringing your reservoir to the tipping point. Your symptoms are real and debilitating, but they are just the alarm. They are communicating to you that there is a problem, but the problem will never be solved by flooding them with your attention day after day. You must turn, bravely and boldly, toward the fire. You must walk into your darkest room and turn on the light.

This is JournalSpeak. This is naming.

Take the time. Prioritize yourself. Simply thinking about one's life has proved insufficient in my experience. You have to slow down and write out your "stuff" and the feelings associated with it. The nervous system doesn't ask your opinion or wait for permission to save your life. If it deems your repressed emotional world as a greater predator than your physical pain and anxiety, it will choose the pain every time. So it is your responsibility to send a message of well-being and safety.

Please listen carefully now, as I'm going to tell you some things about you that you may not consciously appreciate. This is JournalSpeak.

You can feel even your ugliest stuff. You can admit your role in your struggles. You can let your guard down and tell the whole story. You can own your mistakes. You can rage to those who may never willingly hear you. You can beg forgiveness you will never receive. No one is listening but you. You are the only one who needs to hear. You are the creator and the destroyer. You have the power to be brave, look yourself square in the mirror, and walk into the fire.

STAY

Nobody relishes sticking around in their darkest rooms to reflect on the things in their lives that have been painful as hell. You may feel inclined to run away from the sensations that arise. Yet essential for healing is staying with our feelings and reflecting on the ways in which we've been shaped and molded by our experiences. The nervous system senses danger because its only means of understanding is the information it receives from us. *Just like we would never run from safety, we would never stay in a place that wasn't safe.* When you stay, feel what needs to be felt, and acknowledge the truths that have been and continue to be, eventually the alarm bell stops ringing. The pain signals subside. It's okay to look. It's okay to pause and be curious. It's safe to be here. Indeed, it's essential.

As we discussed in Chapter Five, resistance comes in many forms, and they are all meant to dissuade you from staying. When you land on something uncomfortable or a situation that feels impossible to control (most are), resistance will stop by to help you. "Eat this!" it will offer. "Drink this! Run this way! Scroll your phone! Watch this show! Go anywhere but here—it's not safe to feel this deeply!"

My love, close your eyes. Hear my voice in your head. Say to that resistant voice:

"I know, honey. I know. You mean so well. You have kept me alive all of these years with your messages of protection. I hear you, I honor you, I thank you. But we have both been confused. Staying with these feelings is actually safer than being sick and in pain. I know this sounds crazy, but I now recognize the truth. Also, sweet self, I can't live this way anymore. Even if you are convinced that I am not safe being with these painful memories and truths, I'm no longer willing to cosign this physical suffering. My body is screaming at me, and I need to listen. The symptoms are just the alarm bell, though; I need to attend to the fire. I need to stay. I can stay, and I will. And you, my nervous system, can stay, too. I am not banishing you. I am inviting you to join me. You can come, but you can't call the shots anymore. I will hear you out, but I won't follow your directives. I am grown, I am strong, and I am in charge."

Initially, it may feel silly to speak to yourself this way, but it works. Over the years, my clients have repeatedly told me, "My body is against me." I think what people fail to realize is that their bodies (and whole Mindbody systems) are their greatest protectors. By staying with your perceived internal lions and tigers and transforming them into domesticated pets, you allow your inner and outer worlds to align. No one is against anyone here. You've just been confused, and you're not confused anymore.

Breathe, stay, feel, surrender. You can be here. Everything you want is waiting for you.

RELEASE

Let's review some inconvenient truths about release: Release cannot be willed. Release cannot be chosen. Release is not possible when forced. In truth, trying to force it only impedes it. Release, in all its glory, is the result. It's the result of allowing, naming, and being brave enough to stay. As you live these practices, release will naturally follow. In these moments, you will feel the pain fade and your spirits rise. You will sense the lightening of your burden, physically, mentally, and emotionally.

I have lived much of my life resisting and withholding. I spent my childhood constipated. I clenched my teeth when I slept regardless of the nightguard. My anxiety manifested in myriad ways, from trouble swallowing to unrelenting insomnia. I am not a natural releaser, so take it from me, this process I'm teaching you is the way out. I wish I could wave my magic wand and offer the release you are desperate for, right at this moment. But the only way out is through, and the ANSR is your road map.

As I began to live this process long before it had a name, I saw changes in myself that proved its efficacy. My digestion regulated. I stopped getting headaches that I'd always attached to jaw tightness. I could calm my anxious thoughts, and I found sleep. I often contemplate the adage "Without your health, you have nothing," and it rings especially true for those of us who have lived without a healthy body as a partner. I revere this work, even in the struggle, because it has given me the vigorous companion I've always longed for. The relief this method offers needs to be felt to be believed.

Best of all, the life-altering pain you've endured is the biggest (yet littlest) part of the equation. What does this mean? It means that you thought overcoming physical torment was the ultimate objective here, but what you'll discover is that it was simply the doorway to an existence you'd not even considered. Your whole life awaits! A pinprick of light is all that's necessary to expose your current darkness as temporary. The ANSR process will help to relieve your chronic pain and offer you freedom from the hamster wheel of doctors and procedures, but my love, it is so much more than that. Once you begin living in the ANSR, your relationships, self-worth, confidence, ability to handle conflict, and connection to purpose will all start to transform, too. This is the new way of living I keep teasing. It is one that requires tenacity and courage but produces the possibilities and inspiration that have been hidden from you for far too long.

ALLOW YOUR BODY TO BE YOUR PROOF

Prior to this moment in your life, you may not have believed that an emotional exercise could cure a physical condition. Yet once you begin this work, proof of this becomes evident in the form of your body's response: Pain is less prevalent. Stomach issues fail to surface no matter what is eaten. The impending weather front doesn't bring on a migraine. Anxious thoughts don't own you, even when you're dealing with an undeniably stressful situation. The challenge, at the beginning, is to believe that this is possible. This belief is fortified, brick by brick, as you allow your body to be your proof.

Too often people discount their successes by being afraid to believe that indeed *they are the reason for their improvement.* This is a normal defensive reaction. It comes from a deep fear that we don't have agency over our lives, paired with an attendant desperation for good health. Don't allow yourself to be unconsciously baited into this trap. When you make excuses for your tangible results, it can stop improvement in its tracks. When your inner monologues are fueled by fear and lack of confidence based on voices from the past, they can lead you to dismiss even your most hard-fought victories. Let's make a pact that you won't explain away the wins that are the direct result of your hard work. Here's an example of how it might go:

You've been doing the work for a little while, and one morning you're backing down the driveway. You realize that your neck doesn't scream when you turn to look over your shoulder. "It's just a coincidence," you might think. "It's probably because the weather improved," or "It must be the delayed result of that shot I got a couple weeks ago."

No! This is not acceptable!

We are working with brain science, and remember—the brain has little information (other than your conscious input) to know whether you are safe. You cultivate a posture of safety when you intentionally acknowledge that your hard work has yielded results. This intentionally connects the lowering of your overflowing reservoir with the lessening of your symptoms. The brain state of rest and repair is solidified in acknowledging your personal power. You are changing the ways in which your body carries emotional baggage.

As we've discussed quite a bit, there are three facets of my work: Believe, Do the Work, and Patience and Kindness for Yourself. As belief is key to recovery, it is essential to *believe* in what you've done. Your body is offering proof that you have the power to affect your physical and emotional health. Acknowledge this, and you are well on your way. Recall our fave cliché: If you keep doing what you're doing, you'll keep getting what you're getting. We must continually and mindfully embrace the opposite—when you do something differently, you change your life. This mindset is key to progress. In the past, I'm sure you've catastrophized plenty when it came to bad outcomes. I know I have. Today you are challenged to believe in the good.

Let's take a closer look at a common trajectory of consistent work:

After some period of doing the work, you will sense a little change.

Just a little something. Maybe it will be a fleeting moment. You'll be sitting there, or standing there, or reaching for something, or sitting at your desk at work, and for one instant something will shift:

You didn't feel the usual pain you feel at exactly that time of day.

You ate thirty minutes ago, and you haven't had to run to the bathroom.

You've been looking at your computer for over an hour, and not a hint of a headache.

You picked up the laundry bin, and your back didn't jolt you with pain.

Whatever your thing, you will sense a subtle shift, and you will take notice. It may be brief, but you won't be able to deny that it happened. *Hmmmm*, you'll think. And then you'll be tempted to dismiss it as chance. Not today, Satan! Thank that menacing voice for the input, and keep doing the work. Let's keep playing with scenarios (this is fun, right?).

You're on the fifteenth minute of your hike, and you notice that your knee hasn't hurt yet.

You roll over in bed and comprehend that it's five thirty a.m. and you've slept through the night—your shoulder hasn't awakened you in pain.

You've walked your dog three blocks and haven't felt your hip whining at you.

185

You've not even thought of scratching your eczema, and it's ten thirty in the morning.

Then it occurs to you that it is happening. The symptom comes rushing back. "Of course," you think. "I knew I was broken." No! Ignore that fearful nervous system whispering in your ear and keep doing the work.

I can't predict precisely how long it will take in your specific case for your pain to recede so undeniably that you will have no choice but to believe it, but that day will come. The most important thing to embrace is that the proof is in there, waiting for your acknowledgment. As I love to say, the call is coming from inside the house. Pay attention to your body, and don't allow a protective and resistant nervous system to sow seeds of doubt. You are taking charge and rewiring your brain. You are regulating your nervous system through mindset, willingness, intentional effort, and meditation. Believe in the work and you will believe in yourself. And never forget, pain is but an entry point. It invites you in and motivates you to move forward, but there is so much beauty around the bend that has nothing to do with physical distress. As unbelievable as this may sound right now, you will look back on this moment with gratitude one day. You're only at the beginning of what is possible for you.

●

Paul's Recovery from Ankylosing Spondylitis, Cyclical Vomiting, and Crippling Anxiety— Age 62 (Midwestern United States)

I began experiencing lower back pain when I was fourteen. My parents didn't believe me because, as far as they were concerned, no teenage boy has back pain. One day, I couldn't get out of bed. My parents finally accepted that there was a problem, but a good solution was nowhere to be found. I started seeing a chiropractor regularly, but after two years there was little improvement.

It was time to consult an orthopedic surgeon. The tests were performed and films taken. I was diagnosed with spondylolisthesis and had spinal fusion surgery in 1978. It was unsuccessful. I continued to have back pain—mostly muscular pain that would ebb and flow. People were constantly telling me I couldn't do things and I needed to protect my back. As a teenager, I was angry and annoyed about this all the time.

In college I started having issues with IBS. I saw our family doctor, who offered the diagnosis but presented no helpful tools on how to cure it. This condition was embarrassing, and it interfered with my daily life. Many tests later, I went to a GI specialist who put me on a medication that better managed the symptoms, but it was far from ideal. The symptoms would start and stop all the time. I never felt safe. I also began experiencing cracking, tenderness, and swelling in my joints. This scared me, as I thought it could be rheumatoid arthritis. I was too afraid to tell my parents or seek medical attention.

There were many problems at home. My father was an alcoholic and my mother was terminally unhappy. Being the oldest child, I was often the mediator during family disagreements and fights. I was responsible for looking after not only myself but also my parents and other family members. I was going to college and working full time. I know now that this was more stress than anyone in their teenage years should have to manage. When I was twenty-six, my mother was diagnosed with metastatic breast cancer. I spent a great deal of time caring for her, and she passed away when I was thirty years old. Things at home got worse.

I was diagnosed with generalized anxiety disorder after having bouts of insomnia just prior to starting graduate school. I started to see a therapist and a psychiatrist. Similar to my back pain and IBS issues, these episodes would ebb and flow around various life events. I was in an endless loop of the TMS symptom imperative, but I had no idea! As time passed, I started experiencing random joint inflammation—fingers, wrist, knee, and back stiffness. I went to see a rheumatologist and was diagnosed with ankylosing spondylitis (AS). I was frightened about the long-term prognosis. Treatment options were limited, and there was no cure.

I soothed myself by keeping as physically active as possible. This seemed to help manage my conditions and was one of the few things that made me feel good. I had to change my AS and anxiety meds periodically, as it appeared that my body would get used to them and symptoms would flare. Because my bloodwork and other tests were always normal, the doctors told me they would treat me based on how I felt rather than test results (i.e., blood panels or MRIs). This, of course, is the worst-case scenario for a TMSer. I was responsible for my own care, essentially, and I was fueled by fear. I completed countless rounds of physical therapy. Things would settle down and flare again. I was taking more medications and supplements than you could possibly imagine.

One day I woke up and both shoulders were popping and sore. I could not exercise. I was in daily contact with my psychiatrist—we were tweaking medications on the fly. I vacillated between not getting enough sleep and being so sedated that it was difficult to manage daily activities. I had a wonderful wife and felt extremely guilty for putting her through this. I was becoming a foreign person to both her and me. No doctor had any idea what was wrong with me.

I had not hit rock bottom yet. After completing an outpatient treatment program, I started vomiting nonstop for two weeks. I could not eat. I was admitted to the hospital for a week of tests, and sent home (still sick) with a diagnosis of cyclical vomiting. I was prescribed another medication, and after a while it calmed down. The moment the vomiting stopped, my AS flared, but this time in a way that was completely foreign and created more anxiety. I was experiencing shooting pains all over my body. I was diagnosed with fibromyalgia. The doctors also suggested a nerve problem and prescribed gabapentin and Lyrica.

I had to carefully coordinate my care with so many doctors because I was afraid of drug interactions. Managing specialists and appointments was becoming my life, and all joy was completely stripped from my being. I kept asking, "Why is this happening to me? *Is this really what my life is going to be like?*"

Then (finally!) the moment of awakening.

A new doctor, after reviewing my records, hinted about an emotional component to my condition. He didn't say TMS or Mindbody, and he didn't offer any direction except to increase my medications, but something woke up in me. I ruminated on this for a while, but I couldn't make total sense of it. I was already practicing Transcendental Meditation, which I thought was supposed to calm your nervous system—why was I not better, then? I couldn't get it out of my mind that there might be something I had yet to explore.

It was around this time that I was introduced to the work of Nicole Sachs. She was like a kindred spirit, like the sister I never had. Our childhood stories were very similar. She was also diagnosed with spondylolisthesis, but she did not have surgery. Something about the way she spoke with such confidence and authority made me willing to attempt what she was suggesting. I started doing her JournalSpeak work.

To open my mind to this process, I had to look my lifetime of skepticism in the face—of course I was medicalized! I had suffered so much. But the Mindbody connection made sense to me, so I was willing to try. And boy, am I grateful I did! If I hadn't, I might still be on the harrowing ride of pain, symptoms, and doctors.

I learned about acceptance, forgiveness, emotions, boundaries, feelings, community, connectedness, and, most importantly, hope. I must admit there is still so much for me to do and learn—fifty-seven years of neglect cannot be undone in eight months—but I have been given a new lease on life that I value beyond words.

Now I am ninety-five percent better. I have been able to eliminate or decrease so many medications and supplements that I am no longer on a first-name basis with my pharmacist. I'm committed to this work one hundred percent, and I believe that I am on the right path without a doubt. Since I was a young boy I have been exposed to the darkest of the dark, and for the first time I am living in the light at the end of the tunnel.

I do yoga, Pilates, spin classes, swimming, golf, daily Journal-Speak, and meditation. I even restarted playing the guitar and started weight training. I planned a ski trip for early next winter, my first one in five years, and I'm so excited. This all would have been impossible a year ago.

My message to you: Don't give up! Not ever! I'm sure you've heard that recovery is not linear, and I still do have days that aren't quite as I would like. But that's okay with me. I know this is a process, and healing is not a straight line. You will learn this, too. You will learn to speak to your discomfort. You will embrace that you are human, and we are all living it out. Remember, you don't have to spend every waking hour thinking about this work, and "doing more" will not necessarily make you heal faster. Be patient, be kind to yourself, and, most importantly, *know* that you are on the right track.

CHAPTER 11

THE 28-DAY CHALLENGE—PUTTING THE WORK INTO ACTION

A lthough the practice of JournalSpeak may sound simple, doing the work is far from easy—and that's why I come to you again as the expectations queen. As you've gleaned by now, proper expectation setting prepares you most effectively for the road ahead. The hardest part about JournalSpeak is getting yourself to do it—especially at the beginning when your symptoms seem insurmountable. In the preceding chapters we have detailed every kind of resistance, provided examples and guidance to help you become more proficient in letting your core feelings rise, and delineated best practices to encourage consistency. But sometimes you may need a little more help—a structure that builds ritual and keeps you showing up to the page.

THE 28-DAY CHALLENGE

Once I understood the power of JournalSpeak in my own life, I knew I had to find a way to share the practice more broadly. Far too many people were needlessly suffering—and I became passionate and vehement (and borderline desperate) to provide every support possible to help them access this life-changing work. As a natural offshoot of my client base, website, and podcast, I created an interactive Facebook community. The objective was that healing warriors could encourage one another, share wins and challenges, and ask questions. I'll never forget the early days of our group. There were twenty-five people, then sixty. I remember looking at a similar page, seeing 875 members, and thinking, "Wow! Can you imagine if I could get nearly a thousand people discussing this stuff in one place?" Today the group has twenty-five thousand people in active conversation.

While each person's practice is personal, there is much you can learn from others who are endeavoring a similar journey. As they put pen to paper (or fingers to keyboard), they give themselves the freedom to release those buried and perhaps ugly feelings of grief, rage, despair, shame, and fear. I've wiped away tears as I've watched people from all walks of life supporting one another.

It was within this incredible community that the 28-Day Challenge was born.

One day, as I was reading a series of posts about the struggles some members were facing in developing consistency in their JournalSpeak practices, I realized that people required more than just the stories and advice of others to bolster them. People needed a defined path that brought them to the place where their own bodies became their proof. I recalled that over the years, many of my clients saw a noticeable change in their symptoms within four weeks of daily, consistent work. I decided to host a four-week trial—a 28-Day Challenge—to avail community members of the incredible belief that comes when chronic pain relief is undeniably tied to emotional excavation.

I reached out to a group of members who were willing to commit to JournalSpeak (twenty minutes) and meditation (ten minutes) consistently for twenty-eight days. Some people had already started a practice and were looking for ways to expand it. Some were dabbling but having trouble building a regular ritual. Still others found themselves mired in resistance yet eager to forge a path forward. I invited them all to join me. I would do it right alongside them, and we would assess the results together. I knew that if I could help them solidify the habit of a daily practice, they would see just how transformative this work can be.

The first 28-Day Challenge was a resounding success, and the structure became a regular feature in all of my online communities. Now, as thousands walk in tandem, challenges are happening left and right. Independent groups have formed and are supporting each other all over the globe. The confirmation and belief that are stoked by the results of consistent work are rocketing people into the next phase of their healing journeys.

Now it's your turn.

Please understand that this challenge is not about curing yourself in twenty-eight days. I wish it were that easy, trust me. It takes as long as it takes—time, commitment, and consistent practice—to get you to the point where you can be rid of all your chronic symptoms. However, it is a strong catalyst in providing you the opportunity to recognize your body as your proof—to see that your practice and commitment are making a difference. It creates momentum. The inspiration is undeniable.

THE CHALLENGE

Is twenty-eight days enough to move the needle in such a way that it motivates the entire TMS journey?

It turns out the answer is *yes*.

Although recovery is not a straight line and can and will be marked by the natural pitfalls of the human condition, steady work for a solid period of time has proved to be a mighty facilitator for forward motion. The instructions are simple. What's most important is the regularity. And once you see what is possible in a mere four weeks, you will see just how profound the impact of this work can be.

The first step involves taking an inventory of your mental and physical wellness on Day One. I've provided an example worksheet here. Once you've done it, put the sheet of paper away. You won't need it for twenty-eight days.

Then, engage in the practices outlined in this book every day for four weeks. Tick off each day as you complete it. Some people like to keep a physical logbook and Sharpie on hand; others use the calendar app on their phones. It doesn't matter, as long as you commit to the consistency of these twenty-eight days.

Finally, at the end of those four weeks, print out a fresh inventory worksheet. Without looking at your old inventory, map out your symptoms and their severity again.

I know it's daunting, but you are ready. You can do this. You already understand JournalSpeak in all its glory, and have (perhaps begrudgingly) become willing to add meditation to your wellness practice. The challenge invites you to put the pedal to the metal. Your body is standing by, ready to be your proof. Maybe you've been to therapy or kept journals before, but you've not attempted this kind of raw excavation. Or maybe you've experimented inconsistently, and you just need a reboot. Either way, console yourself with the knowledge that when regularly practiced, this work has the power to circumvent the protective function of the nervous system—and allow your emotional reservoir to reduce to healthy levels. This means no chronic pain.

A few key points to remember as you begin your challenge:

1. JournalSpeak is the vehicle for saving your own life—it will not look pretty or polite.

2. JournalSpeak doesn't stay true—some of my most rageful and despairing sessions aimed directly at my family members have yielded immediate and tremendous compassion and love.

3. Throw away your JournalSpeak when you're done. It's like cleaning out your refrigerator. You are getting out gunk that is clogging up the works.

4. Don't forget about patience, kindness, and self-compassion. You are *not* a bad person because you are airing the grievances of an unheard and unseen inner child.

I can't tell you how many times I've walked straight out of my office after doing my JournalSpeak and right into the loveliest interactions with the people closest to me. Even if my partner or children had been the inspiration for the day's excavation, it's never failed to make me appreciate the people I love even more. Once the reservoir is lowered, there is so much free energy to connect and engage. Not to mention, the pain and anxiety melt away. Remember, when there is no present threat from which to protect you, the throbbing and soreness become irrelevant. The brain stops sending them. So replace your fear with curiosity, and allow your deepest places to rage, beg, cry, and kick. It's a gift not only to yourself but to the ones you love.

Here is an illustration of the way JournalSpeak might build on itself as you become more comfortable with its cadence. The unfolding could happen over days or weeks, or in a single session. Don't worry if you don't come to full peace at the end. Eventually, you will. There is no one right way to do this. There is no one way to feel. True readiness is everything, *and readiness is an outcome of—not a precursor to—action.* The following illustrations are written in the first-person language of JournalSpeak as it becomes your second language of truth and healing. They are purposefully brief—just enough to impart the energy of this evolution.

> *LEVEL I:* "*I am overwhelmed with all the things I need to do in a day. Parenting is tiring. Sometimes I wish I could have more time for myself. My family expects so much of me and I always feel guilty if I can't do everything for everybody.*"

> *LEVEL II:* "*My worst problem is my son. He is disrespectful and annoying. Whenever I try to do anything for myself, he demands my attention. He isn't nice to me. The most hurtful part is my husband doesn't stick up for me. He just stands by and allows this! I'm starting to feel really fed up. This reminds me of how it felt growing up with my own father and the way I was ignored. I'm so triggered every day in my own home!*"

> *LEVEL III:* "*This is fucking bullshit. I have been killing myself for this family for years and I've really fucking had it. I can't stand this one more day. I'm done. I'm not doing it anymore. I quit. I'm moving out and they will see how it feels when I'm not here! No one appreciates me.*"

> *LEVEL IV:* "*Wow. It's been a long time since I felt so heard, even if only by myself. These kids—how can I expect them to appreciate me the way I need? Did I appreciate my mom? What is really bothering me? I'm actually mad at myself. I don't demand respect and then I get irritated at others for not providing it. I want everyone to read my mind.*"

LEVEL V: *"I'm experiencing such equanimity lately. Really, I never knew I could feel this way. I can just wear life more loosely. I still get mad, but the rage feels softer now. I'm even able to ask for what I need, and shockingly, my family is willing to give it to me sometimes. The migraines I used to get several times a week are further and further apart. Come to think of it, I haven't had one in days!"*

CHALLENGE YOURSELF

Here are the steps to the 28-Day JournalSpeak Challenge:

DAY ONE: *Take a Day One Inventory using the 1-to-10 scale (with 1 being the least pain/discomfort and 10 being the worst). List all the symptoms you are experiencing, and any other factors you feel are appropriate, including current stressors. At the bottom of the page, write a short paragraph or two I like to call a* mental health snapshot. *It should embody a sense of how it feels to be you on an average day. A sample worksheet is included here, but you can document your symptoms in whichever way feels most natural to you. Once you complete your inventory, put the piece of paper in a drawer, or save the document to your device. You will not need it again for four weeks.*

DAY ONE THROUGH DAY TWENTY-EIGHT: *Do your JournalSpeak and meditation practice—with twenty minutes for writing and ten minutes for self-affirming meditation, as instructed in Chapter Eight—once a day. You can use your lists, try the prompts we've discussed, or simply push to evacuate anything that is renting too much real estate in your head.*

197

DAY TWENTY-EIGHT: Take a new inventory—without looking at what you noted back on Day One. List your symptoms and their severity and provide that mental health snapshot. Now find your Day One Inventory and compare. What has changed, what has stayed the same? Are there life factors that got in the way or helped you? Were there practices that you adopted over the month that evolved your work in a good way, or maybe kept you stuck? Pay attention. This work is yours. For the first time in forever, you are the one in charge of your health. And you are formidable.

The challenge is designed to bring awareness to your personal power. It is designed to center you in the certainty that you can effect change in your physical body and emotional wellness. Your belief in the process will be strengthened when you accept and celebrate the fact that your hard work and consistency created change. The transformations you see are not the result of coincidence or chance. This is you, allowing your repressed feelings to rise. This is you, informing your nervous system that you are no longer served by pain or chronic conditions.

Sample Worksheets for the 28-Day Challenge

DAY 1	SEVERITY (1–10)	LIFE STRESSORS
Symptom:		
Symptom:		
Symptom:		
MENTAL HEALTH SNAPSHOT:		

DAY 28	SEVERITY (1–10)	LIFE STRESSORS
Symptom: Symptom: Symptom:		
MENTAL HEALTH SNAPSHOT:		

Find your electronic copy of the 28-Day Challenge worksheets at www.nicolesachs.com/challenge.

When I launched the first challenge years ago, I was thrilled to see how many participants became aware of the difference Journal-Speak makes. They might not have been cured of their pain or chronic symptoms in four weeks, but by and large they noticed a significant change.

There was the woman from Kentucky whose back pain had often kept her in bed. By the end of the challenge, she was so mobile that she'd taken her dog on a mile-long walk. There was the man from Sweden who had terrible constant psoriasis, who realized at the end of four weeks that he hadn't had a flare-up in days. And there was the woman from Australia whose IBS improved so much that she discontinued her strict elimination diet (that had been causing her misery) with zero ill effects.

These people—as well as the multitude of others who have also embarked upon the challenge—have accomplished something only lived experience can provide: unshakable belief. It is an essential component to the continued regulation of your nervous system and will help you to keep those internal predators at bay as you move forward.

Recovery may not be linear, but it builds. I offer you a toolkit replete with everything you need to take back your agency. You can begin this transformation anytime you want—you just need to pick it up. Oh, and use it.

•

Barb's Recovery from Hip Dysplasia, Sciatica, and Back Pain—Age 56 (Northeastern United States)

We begin our pain journeys feeling unique, alone, and scared. I was no exception. The beginning of my story could be written by thousands of others. My car was rear-ended in an upsetting but non-catastrophic accident. Although I was not badly injured, this incident was followed by back pain I'd never experienced. It usually happened when I was walking long distances. At the time, it was simply an annoyance that I tried to ignore and treat with some Tylenol.

Later that year I was on a ski vacation. Out of nowhere I started experiencing sciatica alongside the back pain. I figured there was something gravely wrong and I began down the medical road. I saw two orthopedists, had X-rays and MRIs, underwent six weeks of physical therapy, and had weekly acupuncture. When none of this touched the pain, I had epidural shots and weeks of daily chiropractic adjustments, steroids, anti-inflammatories, and painkillers.

Nothing worked, at all. The pain was escalating, and alongside it rose the intensity of my fear. I had diagnoses ranging from spondylolisthesis to neck disc degeneration, but these medical labels were always followed by doctors' admissions of "You've probably had this spondylolisthesis for years" and "Your pain levels just don't match what I am seeing on the MRI." The third orthopedist suggested I look at my life and realize that stress can do bad things to our bodies, but I had no idea what to do with this information, so I ignored it.

At this point, I was working from my living room floor—lying on my back with my laptop on my belly. My life as I knew it was over. I started thinking about the hip dysplasia I was born with that landed me in a cast for the first nine months of my life. One of my earliest memories was in a specialist's office in New York City with my parents at four years old. The doctor said I'd need a hip replacement at some point later on, but I could go and live my life as long as my hip "held up." The fear that I had arrived at this inflection point gripped me.

I had lived for forty-five years with no limitations. I was an extremely active, physical person. I prided myself on having gone to the gym daily at five a.m., a practice that began when I worked at a Nautilus gym in college. I ran mud races, hiked long distances, skied, biked, and skydived. My husband is an ultramarathon runner, and our lives had revolved around traveling to anywhere he could participate in races. I would hike trails and explore. We'd been to Antarctica, nine countries, and nineteen U.S. states—all to follow our passions. All of this seemed like a distant memory now. I'd decided that if I was living with the same pain intensity a year from then, life was no longer worth living. All my dreams were over. I couldn't climb Mount Kilimanjaro, I would never walk the Appalachian Trail, and my plans of all future travel with my husband were crushed. Life had nothing for me if it was a life with this much agony. I was not able to sit or drive anymore; how could I go on?

I had a copy of *Healing Back Pain* in my attic. In 1999, I'd heard Howard Stern interview Dr. Sarno and bought a copy for my then-husband who had chronic back pain. He never read the book (and still has chronic pain), but I held on to it for no particular reason other than it was a new book that'd never been read. You can't just throw away a new book!

In my desperation, I crawled up to the attic and found it. I devoured the eighteen-year-old copy, and I knew that *this was it*. I'd tried every other medical option, and nothing helped. This TMS diagnosis was my last chance to see the pain in a new way, and hopefully I could banish it. I tried to adopt a TMS mindset, but I didn't know exactly how to help myself. It was really hard—I steadily got much worse before getting better. My anxiety increased tenfold. I was losing weight because I had no appetite. I became obsessed with finding out everything I could about TMS and located a TMS physician who confirmed my diagnosis and recommended a psychotherapist in my area who would help. On my first visit with the therapist, I poured my heart out about my life's stressors and emotional pain. He was kind and attentive and helped me recognize some places that needed a deeper dive. Still, I wasn't seeing the shift in pain that I needed to feel confident.

Then I found Nicole. First, it was her YouTube videos. I lay there on the floor feeling like she was talking to me and me alone. The fact that she had the same physical diagnosis in her back also helped further the connection. I read everything she published online, signed up for her online course, and started to JournalSpeak.

Around that time, I also recognized that I was obsessing with healing and reaching in too many directions in desperation. I knew in my gut that I had to simplify. I decided to scale back to just the things that felt right. I would read only Dr. Sarno and Nicole. They felt like the most basic and true resources. Nicole's was the only strategy I would use to rid myself of pain, and I focused on that. I ignored all others while I did her online course, and continued to JournalSpeak every day. I was also seeing the psychotherapist every week, but the content of my therapy sessions always came from the discoveries I made in my JournalSpeak.

I am a type T personality to a T (this is an inside joke for us in the TMS community). It means I am extremely competitive, high achieving, I never say no (no boundaries), and I put everyone's needs and feelings before my own; I am a giver and a goodist. Through all the self-discovery, I realized how many of my thoughts had centered on beating myself up for not being good enough. This had gone on my entire life.

I required structure, and I needed to feel like I was doing something to gain some self-esteem in the process. The 28-Day Challenge captured my competitive nature. I did the challenge twice in a row and realized when I measured my progress that I was solidly moving forward. On the Facebook group, I posted my progress, and when others confirmed that I was moving in the right direction, it was so uplifting. My life was changing. By this time, I was back at work, able to sit and drive, and my anxiety was gone. I was getting sleep every night.

One very important component that was critical for me was to stop caring about when the pain would leave. For so many months I'd kept looking to the future, urgent to be rid of my pain. I discovered that this was an absolute block to eliminating it. I had to detach from the expectation. I had to remove the power the pain had over me. I had to not care whatsoever if the pain was there or not. It was only then that it started to melt away. I know now that this worked because the nervous system can't release the pain when it's still receiving a message of fear. My acceptance practice gave it permission to release me from that protection.

I am writing to you from the perspective of having *proof* that my pain is of Mindbody origin. I offer my story as a little piece of this proof to take with you. I am a changed person. I have traveled down deep into my most hidden places and seen the ugly and the beauty. This has resulted in subtle, small changes that have been a series of mini miracles. It all begins and ends with love.

Many other symptoms have resolved along the way without me even intending to get rid of them. This was even more proof to me that the symptom doesn't matter—if you empty your overflowing reservoir of repressed emotions, your body can settle into harmony.

I no longer have bouts of what I used to think were gallbladder flares, no more allergies to any food or animals (this one still blows my mind), no constant anxiety. The Reynaud's syndrome that flared every winter has been gone for four years now, as have many other minor symptoms of the overflowing cup. I still have a body that occasionally pokes me with a prickly nudge of some sort or another, and in these moments I make time to JournalSpeak consistently. I even do the challenge when I need to. Invariably, the symptom disappears as quickly as it came.

We all have emotions that show up in our bodies as disease, pain, skin conditions, stomach stuff, or any other number of medical diagnoses. The list is endless. The most important thing to recognize is that no matter what it is (once you've been checked out for serious structural illness), it is coming from your brain and nervous system's reaction to your unfelt emotions. Call it your subconscious mind, your id, your inner child; the label doesn't matter here, either. Just understand that your emotions are a living component of every cell of your human body. I need to be of healthy, balanced mind *and* body—they are one.

Today, I am working and working out, and I continue to travel the world with my husband. I live every day as my authentic self. I love who I have become. My pain was a teacher and a lesson I will never stop learning for as long as I am blessed with this human experience. There will be future pains, because I have a human body and life is about feeling deeply, but I say, "Bring it on!" I have the awareness and the tools to see clearly, so when that next message comes from my Mindbody, I will listen, and I will love myself through it.

PART III

UNLEARN TO RELEARN

REPARENT: REHAB-ING YOUR RELATIONSHIP WITH YOURSELF

CHAPTER 12

SELF-COMPASSION AND ACCEPTANCE AS ESSENTIAL TOOLS

B y now, you know that most chronic conditions originate from a dysregulated nervous system. Your brain is working overtime to protect you from the overflowing reservoir by sending pain signals (or chronic disease flare-ups), alerting you that it's time to "rest and repair" yourself. So as we continue together on this path to enduring wellness, there are essential practices that will not only ease the burden of the journey but stop extra volume from being deposited in the form of self-criticism, inner loathing, and desperation to change "what is." Think, for a moment, about the importance of energy in any given situation. The energy you bring can either inflame or soothe, and being aware of this truth is more important than ever when approaching chronic pain recovery.

Envision your daily JournalSpeak practice as the bailing out of a sinking boat. You have your proverbial ladle, which allows you, scoop by scoop, to make sure your emotional reservoir doesn't spill over. Remember, this reservoir is filled with unacceptable emotions that will cause the brain to send symptoms when it bubbles over. To this end, it is essential to focus, in every phase of our lives, on keeping the contents of that beaker as low as possible. This leveling may feel exhausting, but please comfort yourself that you are exactly where you need to be. Being human is hard no matter how you slice it, so we aim to focus on the kind of hard that actually moves us forward. In the world of "what hurts vs. what hurts worse," living in pain and chronic anxiety are on one side of the scales, and living this work is on the other. We want to put our energies in the right place. So how do you cultivate the dynamic of calm and peace that's so essential in rewiring your brain?

I have found a powerful answer to this question in the practices of self-compassion and acceptance.

How does it feel to hear those words? Do you reflexively balk at the thought of concepts that may feel like a waste of time or even a show of weakness? If so, I hear you and I get it. You're in good company. As we've touched on, we are a society of "suck-it-uppers." We oppose vulnerability. We tend to dismiss the importance of self-compassion. And we erroneously equate acceptance with agreement, rendering us resistant to the profound relief it offers. I know that accepting a situation for "what it is" feels like you are releasing your desire for it to change, but this is not accurate. In fact, it is the exact energy that keeps a situation from changing at all. We will work together, here, to help you understand the difference.

As we've done consistently together regarding other confusions that have been ingrained in us around health, let's partner to turn *all* of our misplaced thinking around. Self-compassion and acceptance are as integral as anything else I am teaching here. This is, indeed, incredibly exciting stuff. There are two reasons.

First, your number one goal is to be free of chronic symptoms, however they are manifesting for you. When you are being self-compassionate instead of judgmental, there is far less content being dumped into your emotional reservoir on a daily basis. It's impossible to overstate the ways in which hating on ourselves in its many forms contributes to flares in chronic symptoms. The practice of acceptance carries the same weight. When you spend time and energy resisting the "givens" of any situation, you are only swimming against the current. Opening to this fact will free you, incredibly, to make progress. Don't worry—I will provide precise tools to move you into this state of equanimity.

The second reason for embracing these essential practices is so profound it's hard for me to find the right words for its importance. As you work through this program, my loves, your pain will go. You'll see. But as I mentioned in our discussion of the ANSR, pain is the littlest, biggest part. Sure, when you are suffering physically, it's impossible to focus on anything else. But once the pain begins to subside, *these practices* will transform your relationship with yourself. The self-talk generated within them will reparent the sweet and suffering little kid who didn't get what they needed to emotionally thrive. When you hear person after person fall to their knees in gratitude on my podcast, thanking the pain for the ways it's invited them to see the world in new and transformative ways, self-compassion and acceptance are the heart of what they're talking about.

LIFE SEEN THROUGH A GENTLER LENS

Those of us with TMS naturally do a lot of fighting. This is not to say we are an angry or violent set. In fact, we are quite the opposite. Many of us are the kindest, most easygoing, people-pleasey folks around. The fight is internal. We don't give ourselves a break. We think, think, think, all the time. *Did I do that thing wrong? How did I come off in that conversation? Am I good enough to be here? Am I healing quickly enough?* We are vigilant, always on the lookout for how successful or unsuccessful we are, how everyone might be perceiving us, how we may be "in trouble" or screwing it up, or

how we are uniquely flawed. I label this as *fighting* to bring attention to the energy it creates—the opposite of what we need to
regulate our nervous systems and heal.

This internal battle is not only about self-worth or our perception of *personal* success and failure. We maniacally want other
people and situations to do and be as we wish. It makes us feel
safer. We want our partners to read our minds, our children to
make better choices, and our career opportunities to be tailored to
our dreams. And this battle happens all between our ears! Sure,
from time to time we lose it and tell people how to behave, but
much of this furious "longing for different" is internal. It eats at us
from the inside. We are desperate for the world to conform to our
wishes and standards.

This is the human condition. You (and I) may be living in the
midst of the mess, but we also get to choose how to manage it.

Life can be experienced through one of two lenses: love or fear.
This is not a new conversation, but one that is especially crucial
here. When you look at your existence through the lens of fear, you
anxiously need things to be a certain way, whether it's in regard to
yourself or others. You continually scan your world for problems,
and when you find them—which you always will—you get stuck
on what *should* be. Not only does living through the lens of fear
require a ton of emotional repression (as life is never exactly as you
wish), but it creates resistance to the natural process of healing.

The lens of love, in contrast, is gentle. You acknowledge that
life is constantly changing, and human beings are evolutionarily
wired to ebb and flow. When you can learn to "wear life loosely,"
as you'll hear me say, you allow people and situations to be as they
are—rather than how you'd have them be. In this process, your
nervous system no longer has to react so defensively to every stressful situation. The idea of embodying such a manner of living may
feel challenging, but to stop banking repressed emotions into your

reservoir, you must be intentional about the way you behave and think.

Looking at life through a lens of love requires paying attention to how you talk to yourself. I spent years thinking it didn't matter how urgently I lived, how much I shit on myself, or how longingly I wished for people and things to be different than they were. I was wrong—and it left me scrambling to manage symptoms that I didn't need to have in the first place.

In the first several years of my own TMS journey and teaching this work to others, I understood that the road to healing is paved with trust in the process and doing the work to reveal one's repressed emotions. It was only over time, and practicing with suffering people around the world, that I realized how important it is, also, to focus on self-compassion. I watched people get stuck. I observed their frustration and confusion. I realized that it's a slow road to recovery when you are hating on yourself all the time. It's a "two steps forward, three steps back" kind of situation.

Inherent to so many of us in the TMS community is the relentless assault of the inner critic, informing us all the time about how we're screwing it up. It calls our worth and abilities into question. This is old language cultivated over many years of shaming—external and eventually intrinsic. It might have originated under the influence of your father, your mother, your sibling, your teacher, your coach, or a bully at school. As you've grown, it has begun to speak in your own voice. The inner critic's arguments are convincing, and its judgmental declarations dump much rage, shame, grief, terror, and despair into the reservoir. Disarming this menace begins with awareness. Its inner dialogue is so unconscious, we often fail to notice it's happening. Why is it so wily and effective? The answer is rooted in survival.

Consider the concept of perfectionism. I've spent much of my life beating myself up for not being perfect. This certainly has ties to my critical father, but I think it goes deeper than that. Many of us embody perfectionism as a defense mechanism, having used it as a shield during childhood when few things were under our control. If I were just shiny enough, maybe it would ease the frightening and painful aspects of my life that felt so unbearable. I've worked with many clients who've reported that internalized pressure to be flawless began as children, when it felt like it could help them survive abuse, neglect, addiction, and chaos in the family. I know this is true for me.

Self-compassion means treating ourselves with the same kindness and caring we would offer a suffering loved one, friend, or even a stranger. Dr. Kristin Neff, a researcher at the University of Texas at Austin who is well-known for her work on self-compassion, highlights an indisputable truth: We speak in much kinder tones to others than we do to ourselves. When others are hurting, we rush to their sides with empathy and support. When we are hurting, we reflexively look for where we have failed: *It's my fault. I should've known better.* This self-talk can be relentless and toxic. Whether or not we are to blame, the inner critic's voice tends to be the loudest.

Perfectionism, although born of survival, can be amended within the container of self-compassion. If you take a closer look, perfectionism is not honorable or admirable. It's not striving for the highest standards out of love for self or others. Perfectionism is the relentless scanning of your life's landscape, constantly looking for where you screwed up. It's an endless cycle of judgment and ridicule. Because life is a choice between what hurts and what hurts worse (sick of me yet?), I offer you a choice: Continue with your embattled perfectionistic ways (which are directly attached to pain), or lay down your weapon and rewrite survival as giving yourself a break. In chronic pain recovery, here's a spoiler: It hurts worse to stay stuck in impossible standards and self-criticism. Your progress will be limited. The reservoir cannot sustain such input, and the nervous system will not relent if it deems you unsafe. Alternatively, when we quiet the beast and stop disparaging ourselves, it receives the message of safety it so sorely needs to release your pain.

Maybe you've heard this adage batted around: "If hating yourself were going to work, it would've worked by now." Once you accept this concept, self-compassion replaces perfectionism as the act of survival. It saves you in moments of tremendous panic. It rewrites relationships where you previously found yourself constantly defensive and raw. And, most importantly, it's an indispensable tool in relieving your chronic pain, as the reservoir need not contain the inner critic's constant derision. How to practice self-compassion? It's simpler than you might realize. Simple, but not easy, as I tend to say. That's okay, you can do it. We can do simple but not easy things.

We begin with awareness: *I'm noticing that I'm beating myself up right now.*

Great, you are awake. Now pause. Breathe. "I have a choice. I can speak to myself differently. I'm learning that it's in fact essential to do so. I am willing to be a little uncomfortable—this change in self-talk goes against my habitual way of being." And then speak again—this time, with care and kindness for the most important person in your world, you. Remember that everyone suffers, and you are not alone. Consider that you are only hurting yourself by slinging the second arrow. The first arrow may be the mistake you perceive yourself to have made. But the second arrow is your self-talk around it. Choose kindness—because this means you are also choosing freedom from chronic pain.

"I feel terrible. I feel like I screwed up, said the wrong thing, lost my temper, made a mistake, did a poor job, et cetera. I'm sad. Am I going to be accepted? Loved?"

"I might feel like I messed up, but I'm not going to go down the road of shame and blame. I am a person who is hurting right now. That's okay because everyone hurts. I can choose to be gentle with myself right now."

Now go. Do a little caring thing for yourself. Take a walk in nature. Feel the sun on your face. Draw a hot bath. Call a friend you miss, and connect with love. Do it, and watch how you flourish and grow. This may feel silly or unhelpful at first, but resist the urge to heed that old voice. This is the silly and unhelpful stuff that is going to change your life. It has profoundly changed mine. No kindness is ever wasted.

ACCEPTANCE VERSUS THE CLOCK

Urgency to heal is one of the biggest barriers to recovery. This is because it engenders so much fear. This is understandable. Many of you have gone through hell before arriving here. You've been to every doctor and specialist, tried every treatment and medication, done elimination diets and exercise protocols, moved back home to have family take care of you, even moved house to try to evade environmental toxins . . . all to no avail. Of course the need to feel better feels urgent. How could it not?

As you start to do your Mindbody work and master the tools you need to heal, I can understand that you want them to work as soon as humanly possible. You want it done *now*. Unfortunately, these kinds of panicked feelings are a real obstacle to progress. Acceptance of the brain science and a gentle attitude that sends a message of safety to the nervous system are key. To arrive at this state of mind, I think it helps to first unpack the way we naturally view success and progress. It affords us the necessary perspective to combat your reflexive urgent thinking.

We've already discussed how watching the clock is a form of resistance. Let's unpack it further.

Many of us envision time linearly. We move through our lives, executing tasks, checking off calendared meetings and events, and going through the motions. Our default setting is this trancelike state of forward motion, often lapsing into anxiety and sending messages of distress to the nervous system. This can be so automatic; I know it has been in my life. Measuring myself became synonymous with self-worth. I walked through my days constantly checking in on myself. "Am I better than yesterday?" "Am I keeping pace with the person to my left, my right?" "Is there more I can do?" *"Am I even doing it right?"*

Remember, desire to be different than you are translates as fear to the nervous system. You are immersed in a battle between what is authentic and what is acceptable. It is only natural that fear will arise. And, as you now understand, fear is one of the major drivers of TMS. When you feel desperation to be better, faster, more accomplished, or "done," you may find yourself in an endless loop of anxiety and pain. This brand of urgency is present in much of daily life for many of us, but never is it more pronounced than in the TMS healing trajectory. It's so natural to want to watch the clock and create a mental timeline that ends in "better."

It's essential that you understand that this is not the way it works. If you don't continue to remind yourself of this, your brain will lapse into fearful vigilance without your permission. We must redefine the way you identify progress. We must drop into a richer truth, one that has always been true but perhaps was shrouded from view by Disney movies with happy endings or Instagram delusions about other people's perfect lives. The reality is that life is cyclical. We have good days and bad. There is no place to arrive, and no definition of success greater than being present and feeling peace.

215

I know that there are significant markers in life. Milestones, achievements—and they are worth celebrating! But the desire to arrive at "happiness" or "be done" with suffering can keep you stuck as you make your way along the healing path. Instead, it's vital we redefine what it means to ascend. Acceptance is embracing that we are never, ever, going to live in a place that is *all better*. This is true not only for people with chronic pain or conditions. It's true for every one of us. This is the human condition. There is a cure for chronic pain, as chronic pain is an epidemic of fear, but there is no cure for being human. Life is hard and painful, and there is no such thing as a perpetual state of happiness. But that is okay! Thankfully, the same goes for states of sadness, or hopelessness, or anger. Living exists in moments, and we can open ourselves to many more joyful ones when we view them from the right perspective.

There will be rough days and days of ease. Although it will not always feel comfortable, rest assured that progress will be apparent if you can adjust your lens to that of acceptance. The path of change is not direct, and neither is your experience of being a person in the world. Your lessons are not learned once. Transformation happens over time, with setbacks and course corrections. We all must encounter situations again and again, in slightly different forms, before we start recognizing patterns and tuning our responses. In terms of moving beyond chronic pain, in which the primary job is to send a message of safety to the nervous system, you are tasked here to reframe your expectations around what it means to be well.

Buddhism teaches that all suffering derives from the "clinging of mind." We grasp at states of being, wanting them to remain—permanently—when we feel good. This fixation causes us to struggle, as we equate safety with achieving a certain outcome. The truth of the matter is that the only constant in life is change.

Far too often, when we get even a whiff of instability about an outcome we seek, we find ourselves plunged into a pit of despair and doubt. In the fear-driven linear view of healing, one win should lead to the next in chronological order, right? And if there is any sort of backsliding, it feels like failure. This is a delusion that causes great distress. The truth, in case you need to hear it one more time:

Recovery, from anything, is not a straight line.

Rather than a treacherous climb from the base of the mountain to the summit, it is a journey of concentric circles winding its way to the top. There is a natural urgency that comes with being in pain and discovering a new healing modality. You want to master it and move on. Yet this is not a reality in this work or in any method that promises an enduring solution. Let's sit with this mountain metaphor. It may soothe your trembling mind that is desperate for permanent outcomes to feel safe. I know mine can quiver like a panicked child when I'm trying to embrace something new.

Take a moment and conjure an image of a hike up a scenic mountain. The trail wraps gently around, revealing different landscapes at every turn. This hike represents your healing journey. On some days the terrain will be rocky and the weather rough; on other days the sun so bright and stunning you will need to shield your eyes to see—and every condition in between. As you move up and around the mountain, you feel yourself ascending. Maybe there is a lightness in your step, your pain is lessening, and you sense ease on the path. Wonderful! But then you round the bend, the weather turns, and the trail becomes more treacherous. You have a flare in pain, or the symptom imperative takes hold and you experience sensations of discomfort in your body.

As this struggle feels familiar, you're tempted to say to yourself in frustration, "How can I be here again, right back where I started? How can my back pain be with me again? I thought that was over— I passed that miles ago!"

Pause. Turn around, and look back and down. Take note that the place you stand is not *exactly where you've been*. You are better, more able, less burdened. Your mindset is different; you know what to do when pain knocks at the door. You are, in fact, ascending. As you allow your body to be your proof again and again, you will see that you are changing. You are not having "the same pain experience." You're not lost in it anymore. You're not mired in your story or trapped in your patterns. You're exactly where you need to be. *This is acceptance of the process.* It generates a rewriting of a lifelong story of success and failure and gives you the freedom to widen your lens.

No one is psyched about a pain flare, IBS symptoms coming back for a return visit, or a migraine after months of being symptom-free. And you don't need to be okay with feeling a backslide in your recovery. But think of it this way: The slower you go, the quicker you get there. This means that when you practice acceptance and do not panic that your progress is "ruined," your nervous system will regulate much more quickly each time, and the flare will ease.

This poem by Portia Nelson has always beautifully embodied the ascension metaphor for me. If you think of each challenge in your journey as taking on the route she describes as you hike up your own mountain, you will naturally calm the imperative to heal that breeds so much fear and resistance. Epiphany is possible when you are awake, aware, engaged, and present. It is in this state that you are able to take responsibility for your reactions, calm your need for things to be different, and open yourself to "wearing life loosely."

"An Autobiography in Five Short Chapters"
BY PORTIA NELSON

I.
I walk down the street.
There is a deep hole in the sidewalk. I fall in. I am lost. I am
helpless.

It isn't my fault.

It takes forever to find a way out.

II.

I walk down the same street. There is a deep hole in the sidewalk. I still don't see it. I fall in again.

I can't believe I am in the same place. It isn't my fault.

It still takes a long time to get out.

III.

I walk down the same street. There is a deep hole in the sidewalk.

I see it there, I still fall in.

It's habit. It's my fault. I know where I am. I get out immediately.

IV.

I walk down the same street. There is a deep hole in the sidewalk. I walk around it.

V.

I walk down a different street.

AN EXERCISE FOR RADICAL ACCEPTANCE

There is no more exhausting experience than needing things to be as you "require" to move comfortably through life. The antidote for this is radical acceptance.

The first step in embracing radical acceptance is awareness—seeing ourselves for who and what we are. If our perfectionistic, controlling, and self-critical tendencies were sown as survival techniques during painful times, we begin by honoring them for saving our lives. There is no part of you that is wrong, bad, or by mistake. You have done the best you could with what you've been given thus far. Now that you know better, as Maya Angelou so sagely told us, you can do better.

A TRANSFORMATIVE EXERCISE

I often reference author Danielle LaPorte's query in the book *White Hot Truth*: "Can you imagine not craving to be any different than you are right now? Because here's the sacred paradox: Transformation begins with the radical acceptance of what is." The first time I read this passage, the words immediately resonated. Danielle is right. There is no transformation possible when we are fighting everything and everyone. I realized that if "transformation begins with the radical acceptance of what is," then acceptance, the salve for so much inner struggle, is predicated on uncovering *what is*. You do this by taking the time to observe your environment and identify the people, situations, and issues that may be keeping your reservoir filled to the brim.

Start by making a list of all the things in your life that you wish were different. It could include aspects of your personality, your children in all their glory, your partner, your lack of a partner, your job, your financial situation, or whatever else you spend time wishing would change. Your list can contain anything that might possibly cause conflict or struggle as it exists today.

Then, for each item, pick up pen and paper (or laptop and keyboard), and describe it *as it is*. Begin by pretending that you are a court reporter, unemotionally describing the situation as if you simply had to see the whole picture in words. Here's an example of how to begin:

Topic: My Type A Sister

My sister is a perfectionist. She has a certain way of doing things and has difficulty understanding why anyone would do anything differently. This can make our get-togethers very stressful. She not only comments on my house, my partner, and my children—she offers unsolicited advice on what to do so my life can look more like hers. The thing is, I don't want my life to be exactly like my sister's. She puts so much pressure on herself to be a certain way—and for things to look a certain way. Who has the energy for that? It makes it so I don't want to spend as much time with her because I feel like she's always criticizing me and the people I care about most. When I try to tell her that I like things as they are, she makes this pinched face like I'm full of shit.

As emotion arises, let it come:

I honestly think she's full of shit. I know her life isn't perfect. No one's life is. Her kids can be just as obnoxious as mine. If you take away that Pinterest veneer, she's struggling just like the rest of us. I just wish she could be honest about it instead of always picking at me and my family. I don't want to fight with her—and I don't want to cause drama at family events—but I am getting angrier and angrier. I don't want to have to deal with her.

Like your regular JournalSpeak practice, continue writing for a full twenty minutes. Set an alarm to make sure you are giving it your full attention—and even if you feel stuck, keep writing. The goal is to document *what is*.

When you are finished, read it slowly and without resistance. *This is what is.* Sure, you might prefer it to be different, but that doesn't change the truth of the moment. Fighting it is pointless and will only cause you frustration and more volume in the reservoir. As spiritual innovator Byron Katie is known for saying, "When you argue with reality, you lose—but only 100% of the time." All you have to do is read it over, and say to yourself, "Okay. This is what is." Breathe deeply. Let out a slow and longer exhale. Here we are. This is *what is*.

221

Now it's time to accept it.

Acceptance is about making a decision. It is laying down your weapon of "wishing it were otherwise" and knowing that it hurts worse to keep fighting what is. When you feel resistance in the form of a tantruming mind that equates acceptance with agreement, console yourself with the fact that acceptance sends an immediate message of safety to your nervous system. Few people have any idea of the amount of energy they spend on panicking that things are not as they "should be." When you pause and gaze upon *what is* without needing to change or control it, you are protected from your own directives to fix, save, or manage the problem. Your whole system rests and resets. I cannot overemphasize the power of this posture. Try it, and you'll see.

ACCEPTANCE AND SELF-COMPASSION

This radical acceptance exercise is also a great tool for accessing self-compassion. When we're not inadvertently fighting a situation to try to make it different or "better," there is room for perspective. Maybe your child won't make good decisions, your partner won't stop drinking, or your finances are not where you want them to be. But today, that is simply what is. You would like it to transform, and you can do everything reasonable in your power to live in the solution, but beating yourself up about the current status won't help. Instead, it will cause you pain and block the vitality necessary to envision and create a different picture. Self-compassion lives in the space of acceptance. It lives in the place where you don't need anything to be different, just for this moment. You are enough, and so are others. It may sound hokey or trite, but this posture is fertile ground for neural rewiring.

We are all part of a human collective who suffer, each in our own way. You are not alone, unique, or hopeless. This may seem obvious or banal, but I've found over years of practice that when people fail to pause and acknowledge this, their healing is significantly decelerated. Acceptance and self-compassion quiet the inner critic and provide the impetus to move through the weeds of your childhood trauma, daily triggers, and long-held personality traits that have been keeping you stuck.

Because transformation begins with the radical acceptance of what is, as you achieve more and more moments of this brand of acceptance, you open the door to change. *And change, you will.* Over and over again, I watch the most tragic cases of debilitating chronic pain totally resolve. I witness relationships mend. I see anxiety and depression lift. Whole lives move from small, stuck spaces to expansive and vibrant landscapes.

THE STRUGGLE IMPERATIVE

Another reason that self-compassion and acceptance will change your life is because of the endless hamster wheel of angst I like to call the struggle imperative. You know by now about the symptom imperative, Dr. Sarno's description of chronic symptoms moving around the body as you challenge the nervous system's protective stance. The brain's desperation to divert you from your overflowing reservoir causes the cycle many TMSers know well: Once you find relief for your back pain, the headaches come on. After you do the work to relieve the headaches, stomach issues may begin out of nowhere. And so on, and so on. This trajectory doesn't happen to everyone, but it is prevalent enough to take note. This can be a frustrating dance—but, as we discussed earlier, it's a sign that you are dealing with TMS and not something structural. It also means you are on the right path with JournalSpeak and meditation. When chronic pain or anxiety is on the run, it means it's on its way out of your system for good.

I came up with the "struggle imperative" one morning as I (with horror) realized I was doing it to myself. It's like the symptom imperative, but instead of symptoms moving around, it's your worries, fears, and "problems." Once you've dealt with something big and feel the emotions surrounding it begin to wane, all of a sudden something else pops up in its place, draining your emotional energy. This is especially true once you've done enough of this work to get your symptoms to diminish. Instead of feeling the struggles around physical pain, you may suddenly feel angry about local politics, become anxious about your partner's health, or start beating yourself up about your weight.

This is understandable. You've been fighting fires for so long, and the brain innately seeks what it has known before. When you get to a point where you aren't always reacting, space remains. It's the human condition that something else will reflexively rise and take its place. You know what they say: Nature abhors a vacuum. As you find physical relief, your brain will unconsciously look to fill the space your pain occupied with something else. Similar to any other TMS, this process is perceived as protective by your nervous system. Worry and fear launch you "into action," even if that action is just perseverating all night about your son's breakup or your partner's problems at work. This mindset is not helpful, and I don't want you to get involuntarily lost in the loop. We need to stay awake (but not all night long)!

Per usual, awareness is key. The struggle imperative is normal and human, and happens to us all. Self-compassion and acceptance can turn it around. They counteract the reflexive loop of the struggle imperative by keeping you focused on your humanity and authenticity, rather than allowing your brain to take the reins and seek the familiarity of worry and strife. This reduces reservoir input, so you can stop working so hard to bail out.

Through these practices, you will be opened to experiencing

life through the lens of love. Your body will follow. Your vessel will be seaworthy. You will live free from chronic pain, embrace and expand your relationships, and cultivate a tender bond between you and the very most important person in the world. I won't say it again. You know who it is.

●

Claire's Recovery from Pelvic Pain and Vulvodynia—Age 61 (Scotland)

I had chronic pelvic pain for over twenty years with a diagnosis of vulvodynia, which helped *not at all* in providing guidance for recovery. I traveled around the world and sought help in the UK, Australia, and the United States. I tried tons of medications, physical therapy, and attempting to "just ignore it," but nothing provided relief. I became depressed and hopeless. I could go on about the anguish and trauma of spending this amount of time with such a delicate and embarrassing condition, but I would much rather tell you how the years have gone since I was graced with the knowledge of these theories and practices. As Nicole says, I want to help you to "live in the solution."

My turnaround began when I encountered a physical therapist whom I had flown overseas to consult. He was the first person to ask me about how things were going in my life. At the time, my father had recently passed away after a short illness, and I'd been totally unprepared for it. He suggested I might benefit from seeking emotional and mental support.

After a few months of resisting the PT's recommendation, I set up an appointment with a counselor. I figured I could get help coping with my catastrophic thoughts around how this chronic pain was ruining my life. After a short time of getting to know one another, she gently suggested that I look into Dr. John Sarno. I read *Healing Back Pain* in one day and saw myself on every page, particularly in the typical TMS personality type. I'd always especially wanted to be good, well-liked, and perfect. I'd shame myself greatly whenever I made a mistake.

I threw myself into reading everything I could about TMS. I was pretty sure that this phenomenon was happening to me, but I still had some doubts. This was mainly because at that time most of Sarno's literature was focused on back pain. I am, by nature, a researcher with an analytical mind. It's easy to get caught in a trap of reading and seeking too much. I also tend to compare myself negatively with others who seem to recover (or achieve in general) more quickly. In the beginning, I made all these mistakes.

Looking back on my life, I began to understand that a lot of external factors were contributing to my distress at the time I first noticed the symptoms. I was in a demanding job in a male-dominated environment, I had moved away from home to accept a promotion, and my mother had been diagnosed with cancer. The decades-long pursuit of a cure for my condition was itself traumatic. Recognizing all of this helped further the belief that I had TMS. I made some progress, but although the symptoms lessened in intensity and duration, they didn't go away.

Intellectually, I completely understood that the pain was an expression of my repressed emotions—the fear and meaning I'd placed on my life—but starting to change this was hard for me. I didn't know where to begin. How do you rewrite the screenplay of your entire personality and life's experiences? I decided to start at ground zero with emotions. I had very few skills in even recognizing what I was feeling, and I certainly wasn't able to articulate it. I can laugh now, but at the time it was really tough and embarrassing to say "I don't know" or "Nothing" when my counselor would ask how I felt or what sensations I could identify. It was awkward that, as a grown woman, I couldn't answer such basic inquiries. In retrospect, no one ever taught me how!

I felt stuck until I found Nicole's work in a Twitter post. I liked Nicole's approach because she was so calm and confident, and her connection to Dr. Sarno made it easy to trust her. She was doing something concrete that built on Dr. Sarno's work. I was reinvigorated to heal.

I initially approached JournalSpeak with my usual "good girl" conditioning, wanting to be excellent at it. I was accustomed to getting results from the first effort I put in, but Mindbody work didn't respond the way I expected. I became frustrated when I could not nail this thing one hundred percent and right away.

As I continued to walk the path, I realized I could simply devote thirty minutes to my JournalSpeak practice (twenty for journaling, ten for meditation) and then move on with my day, knowing that the work was done. It helped me to get out of my perfectionistic way. I started to treat JournalSpeak like I would a commitment to an exercise program or learning a musical instrument, where the rewards of practice don't always come immediately. On some days I felt a great release of insight, and on some days I felt nothing at all. But I knew in the long run this didn't matter.

I can remember the day that I listened to Nicole's episode titled "Clara's Story—The Unmet Needs of the Sensitive Child." Previously, I had worried that I couldn't get well, as I regarded my childhood as "good" with no significant trauma, such as death or divorce. My life didn't seem to justify the level of pain I had experienced. A deeper, gentler look revealed a picture of my mother as a very anxious person, and though I know my parents absolutely did their best, they were not armed with knowledge of how to support me emotionally.

I grew up in a time of stoicism, one of being grateful for what you had compared to others and not making yourself the center of attention. It was anathema to ask for your needs to be met. I could see how this had shaped me, and it was freeing. Giving myself permission to sit with these energies of childhood revealed many of my patterns of people-pleasing and conflict avoidance. I had needed them to survive growing up, but now they were making me sick. The self-discovery freed me to change many behaviors. I started speaking up, saying no, and being prepared to live with the consequences. This was far from easy, but in the world of "what hurts versus what hurts worse," there was no question that the discomfort was worth it.

Consistency with the work is key, but I think a better word for it is *persistence*—practice regularly, but not with self-imposed pressure. If you miss a session, don't get lost in self-flagellation. You are doing the best you can.

One of the most joyful and helpful parts of my recovery has been my involvement in Nicole's online communities. I recommend doing the work in concert with other people if you can. It's certainly possible to "go it alone," but for me that was part of the problem. I had to unlearn my stoic tendencies, having always held things close to my chest. I had to challenge my hyperindependence. I feel passionately that being heard and met with empathy and understanding is an important part of healing, especially if you have suffered for a long time.

The symptoms eventually dissolved completely, alongside other things that I realize now were also manifestations of TMS—knee pain, rib pain, chronic postnasal drip. Sometimes things crop up, especially when I put myself under a lot of pressure, but I know what to do.

When I first started as a volunteer moderator on Nicole's Facebook community, I did have a flare-up. I was exposing myself regularly to discussions of symptoms and painful stories there, and it took me a while to work through this and address all the feelings of not being perfect while supporting others. I also had to get comfortable with the experience of people being upset or disagreeing with me. I knew that I merely had more learning to do. I am a sensitive people pleaser who has TMS! Complete freedom in my life must include addressing the way that these qualities crop up in my interactions.

I still do JournalSpeak once a week, and more often when issues and frustrations arise. I consider my practice a form of relapse prevention. If I have a twinge in a tender spot, I have all the necessary tools. I've learned that it is not required to change everything about oneself to be free of chronic pain or symptoms. Our sensitive natures, willingness to help others, and desire to be liked or approved of do not need to be cast out. Many times these qualities can even be desirable, but they need to be understood and perhaps dialed back, making room for other ways to be.

With the pain gone, space has opened up for me to enjoy various passions, including music, running, swimming outdoors, gardening, volunteering, and supporting others doing this work. When I run wearing my T-shirt that says *Ask me how I recovered from chronic pain!*, I love all the conversations that people strike up with me.

Believe in yourself and your capability to heal. Be kind and patient, just as you would for a dear friend who was facing the same challenges. Being in pain for decades is not an impediment to success in this work. I am living proof.

CHAPTER 13

INNER CHILD WORK IS TRANSFORMATIVE

In the history of psychotherapy and "self-help," there has been a lot of discussion of the inner child. Over the years, this concept has become diluted into New Agey rhetoric that tempts people to reject it as esoteric or inaccessible. I used to feel this way. I used to dismiss the whole notion, finding it silly and light. I thought, *We're here to do serious healing! There is no room for pretend play with our internal princesses or finding our toddler bliss.* As is often the case, experience adjusted my sails. I love to be wrong. I cherish the moments when I think I'm so smart and sure, and life smacks me in the face with perspective. Personally, there is no greater relief than knowing that I don't know everything. And so it went, here, with the absolute fucking magic of inner child healing.

INNER CHILD WORK IS ABOUT BEING HEARD

I'd investigated some interesting viewpoints on this kind of therapeutic work, but the profound shift in my perception of inner child theory occurred through personal experience. When my son was in seventh grade, he came home from school and informed me with some sadness (but certainly not despair) that he wasn't invited to the party many of his friends were attending that evening. Then, without much pomp and circumstance, he went about his afternoon.

You would have thought I was hit by a truck. I immediately became highly anxious, fatigued, and unable to think of anything else. I got a dull headache. I replayed the tapes of his childhood, the times he'd struggled socially, the hardships that felt so unique to his sweet little nature. I kept checking in on him (which he found annoying after a bit), and felt a horrible pit in my stomach about his potential inability to be included.

Would he always struggle like this? I couldn't let it go.

The mental and physical reaction I was having hijacked the rest of my day, and when I finally tried to go to bed, I couldn't sleep. The minimal understanding I had of inner child work floated across my consciousness. Desperate and wired, I decided it was time to become curious about this extreme reaction I was having. Who, exactly, was hurting? Was it me, the grown-ass adult who was handily parenting her kids and building a vibrant global practice? Or was it someone else—someone little and far less powerful—begging to be heard? Something felt off. I knew I had to investigate.

I grabbed my computer and opened a blank document, as I do when I am ready to JournalSpeak. Then I paused and found in my mind a mental snapshot of myself in seventh grade. I took a look at her: chubby, new to her school, unsure of her place in the order of things. I could immediately feel the pull of her energy, as if she had terribly important information to share and had been waiting a long time to finally get my attention. Previously, I'd understood inner child work to be about speaking to the little "you" inside, assuring them that you are in charge now and nothing is going to hurt them anymore. In this situation, though, I felt that it wasn't going to heal me to speak to her. She had been waiting patiently, for years, for me to *listen*.

I regarded her, in my mind, with openness and empathy. I felt an old urge to berate her, the way I'd always done when she was me. Drawing on the concepts of acceptance and self-compassion we discussed in the last chapter, I hesitated. Instead of granting access to that critical voice, I decided to look at her with compassion and love. This was not easy, and I struggled against my brain's innate desire to dismiss her as I'd done in the past. But with resolve and intention, I was able to be still and nonjudgmental. I saw "what is," exactly as she was—nothing more, nothing less.

Holding a mental picture of her in my awareness, I took a deep breath and asked her, "What is it like to be you?" I went on: "It's okay, you can tell me. I'm not going to try to make it right, lecture you, or assure you everything is going to be okay when you think it's not. Tell me, what is it like to have your parents, your friends? What is it like to live in your body? I just want to listen. I want to understand how it feels to walk in your shoes."

I put my fingers onto the keyboard and let her speak. She told me of her sadness, her uncertainty, her desperation to be liked. She told me what it was like to live with her mom and dad—their behaviors and decisions. She told me about the bully, Jenny, and how hurtful she could be. She reminded me how awkward it was when her dying grandfather lived in her house. Of course, I knew these stories. But hearing them through her voice was a new experience. It was surprisingly natural to do so, and to send kindness and love as she shared herself with me. The healing was so obvious it made me laugh out loud. I was onto something powerful.

I listened as she spoke. I didn't try to fix or save. At the end, I said, "Thank you for sharing this with me. I am here anytime you want to talk. I really hear you, and I see you. You're not alone in it anymore." As I finished writing and laid my head on the pillow, I knew I had just tapped into something essential. There was a child inside me who had been badly hurting, and by letting her speak and witnessing her pain without judgment or correction, I felt us integrate. I felt at peace. When my attention shifted back to my son, suddenly he was a totally different person from a few hours earlier. Far from devastated, he was strong, handling a tough experience with poise. Equipped with his own strengths and tools, he was doing pretty great. In actuality, I had been overidentifying with my *own inner child*, not with him. I fell asleep that night with ease.

From that day forward, I began to incorporate this brand of inner child philosophy and practice into work with people with chronic pain and anxiety. I also did the exercise regularly myself. As I noted people's overwhelmingly encouraging response, I began to see the application of compassionate listening through Journal-Speak as a powerful tool in transforming our knee-jerk reactions to life's stressors. Triggers can own us without the proper perspective.

What is a trigger, after all, if not a slingshot from the present moment into an unresolved experience of the past?

When a person finds themself violently catapulted into the space of their raw pain and traumatic memories, they have little choice but to react with defensiveness and self-protection. Often this reaction involves a flare of pain or symptoms. You have the power to repair these wounds by witnessing and receiving yourself in ways you'd never had access to while growing up. In doing so, your struggles will find resolution. Your triggers will lose their influence.

When I bring people through inner child work, there is a overwhelming shift in thinking and feeling that comes, at times, instantaneously. Our inner children are often angry and reactive, as they've never been heard. I mean, can we honestly blame them? How would anyone feel in a relationship in which they'd been ignored, dismissed, marginalized, and forgotten? Given this fact, without the proper attention and care, these little shits can pull the strings of our behavior. An inner child practice circumvents this dynamic. There is a tremendous internal appreciation that springs forth ignited merely by your willingness to listen. As your unwanted reactions to life change, you will be both incredulous and relieved. All of this simply by witnessing the distress of the little kid who lives within each of us! This effort has changed me as a parent, a partner, a teacher, and a friend. Just as it has been pivotal in my maintaining vibrant health and ease in the world, so too will it be for you.

Inner child work is also an excellent vehicle for uncovering conflict in your relationship with self and others. Recall that in TMS work, conflict is the biggest catalyst for struggle and confusion. When something is overtly horrible or joyful, there is little TMS attached to it. You are naturally able to label it, feel it, understand it. You may need to come back to traumatizing events again and again to work through them, but when inner conflict is absent, the process is cleaner. This is because it's very hard for human beings to hold two feelings at once (e.g., *I need you, but I don't want you, because you've hurt me*).

Inner child work is helpful because, for most of us, the past is rife with conflict. I am no exception. In many ways, I had great parents. They were loving and supportive, and often my biggest cheerleaders—even my dad. But they were also fraught with their own financial woes, day-to-day stressors, and all aspects of being grown-ups. I know now that one of the reasons my inner sanctum remained unexplored for so long was that my mother couldn't tolerate her own distress over my anguish. As a parent myself, I can really empathize with this. It takes *so much* awareness and education to have the fortitude to override your own discomfort and listen to a child, even if you can't fix things—especially when their suffering makes you feel like a failure.

Whatever your particular childhood experience, your inner child work provides healing in a way that others were not able to offer.

You get to do it for yourself, now, with love and presence. It is a privilege and an honor to listen to your inner children. It is an empowering revelation to unmask your triggers and reverse them. You will gain access to the depths of you, allowing for insights and connections previously obscured. Most pointedly for our work together, you will reduce the repression that leaves you suffering in physical pain.

Let's delve into the philosophy that underlies these practices. It will better help you adopt the mindset for this powerful work. The basic tenets take into account the way we move through the world, floating constantly between the unconscious and the conscious. We are all channeling one of three versions of ourselves at any given moment. When we are feeling unmoored, overwhelmed, anxious, despairing, or discouraged, this is a sign that our inner child is present. Conversely, when we're feeling elevated, peaceful, in gear, and on the right track even though we're not holding the map, we are channeling the higher self. Then there is the middle ground (where we spend most of our time), where we are attempting to manage our lives one way or another, filling in the holes, and doing our best with a forced smile on our faces. This state is when the inner child is doing the "higher self-impression." This is also the breeding ground for much chronic pain and anxiety.

The inner child within us believes "If it were different, it would be better." It is this little one inside that is feeling the displacement, abandonment, loneliness, and discouragement in not having the things that we want. The higher self knows that everything is always changing, morphing from one state to another, and the lesson is in learning to move through adversity with equanimity. It is within this mindset of self-compassion and acceptance that the optimal conditions for healing and wellness reside.

The moment we realize that it is the inner child who is feeling unmoored, we can employ specific strategies to attend to them before they assume the higher self-impression and attempt to manage our days, fill the void, or fix the perceived problem—generating symptoms. When the inner child is heard, they are not trying to direct our lives, which is a relief, because they have no idea what to do. When we access the higher self, we can find peace no matter the circumstance and assist the nervous system in calming chronic issues.

The little kids inside us are angry, sad, and scared. Even though you are no longer a toddler or preschooler having a tantrum, your core reactions to life and the feelings associated with frustration don't change. When grown-up you is enraged and wounded, it's not appropriate to throw a fit, tell someone every single thing you think of them, or walk out of the room in the middle of the conversation. When we get infuriated, embarrassed, and ashamed, we have to repress those feelings to get through the day. This is part of being a civilized adult, but until the inner child is able to be heard, the reflexive bottling up and shoving down has consequences.

For a moment, picture a loving adult whom you know, and then picture yourself at a vulnerable age. It would certainly be impactful to hear them express to you that you are okay, enough, good, and loved. Language like this can heal. Yet now, imagine if they were to drop everything, including their own needs and judgments, and listen to you. Picture a younger version of yourself having their full attention, with no goal other than to make you feel seen and heard. Can you sense the power of that notion? When I've worked with teenagers, I've often heard them say that their most fervent desire is to be known, acknowledged, and heard. Even the best parents can neglect this need in their children, simply because parenting is stressful and requires us to manage so many (often emotional) things at once. This is made even harder when our crafty trauma blocks us from accessing empathy.

Most of us walk around living our grown-up lives—working, dealing with different personalities and life stressors, managing our money, taking care of others. We have no idea that we are living in the space of constant triggers. The moment something touches into the painful wound of not being heard, we can react explosively and inappropriately. Then there is the cleanup after each mess and the resounding side effects. This requirement to pick up after ourselves and others is no longer necessary when you are armed with this powerful tool.

The magic in this brand of inner child work is that it relieves you of unconsciously longing for something you didn't receive. You can intentionally give it to yourself. As you attempt this, you will become aware of the vast landscape of little children inside you who have never been properly heard, and you will revel in your power to attend to them now. You are no longer a little kid. You are no longer powerless and small. What a gift to be the adult that you needed in your youth.

INNER CHILD MEDITATION AND JOURNALSPEAK

The following practice will guide you in finding the right energy for accessing your inner child. Read it to yourself, and then (if you're brave) speak a version of it into a recording device so you can do the practice on your own in the future. Be creative. This is only for you. I like to play meditation music in the background to create an even more soothing atmosphere. This exercise is a powerful portal into the tender world where a lot of healing resides.

Take a deep breath, center yourself, and relax into your body.

Imagine, picture, or pretend that your inner child is standing in front of you. Just take notice of the age they are today, what clothes they have on, how they are wearing their hair. Are they holding anything, do they have shoes on? There is no right or wrong way to do this. You are just becoming aware of how they might appear to you, as it will change from day to day.

In whatever way that feels comfortable, with arms spread and a smile, you might lift them into your arms, or sit on the floor and let them crawl into your lap, or hang out beside a teenage version who needs some space. Tell them how much you love them, and then gently ask, "How are you? Is there anything you'd like to tell me? I just want to know what it's like to be you. I'm fascinated."

Listen without interrupting. There might be a tendency to want to console, or tell them that everything is going to be all right, or explain how you are going to fix something . . . but just listen. You may hear them the way you hear your own thoughts, or they may get emotional and the emoting may come through you. You might just feel what they feel, like an energy. There is no right or wrong. Listen to them until they are complete, and when they are, say, "Is there anything else, love? I want to hear anything you need to say. I'm not going anywhere." Many times you'll find that they want to go back in, to express themselves more fully or to find something deeper. That's okay. Simply listen again without interruption.

This is a tender thing for you to do for your inner child, because so infrequently have they ever been asked to express themselves without interruption—especially when what they were communicating wasn't deemed "polite."

When they are done, completely done, say, "Thank you." Because very, very infrequently in this lifetime have you ever been thanked for fully expressing your emotions. Say, "Thank you. I love you. You're safe. I'm going to take care of everything for you. You can be wonderfully in charge of all the play, but I'm going to take care of the rest. I've got this."

Give them a mighty hug if that feels good. On some days they'll want to skip off and play a game, and on some days, intuitively, they will want to sit beside you and read a book. There is no way it needs to be. The purpose is not to send them away or to make sure you are holding their hand all day. The purpose is to check in with them, so they begin to understand that no matter what they are feeling, you are still going to show up for them. Maybe three days ago they threw a fit, and yesterday they were giggling uncontrollably, and today they are serious and sad. No matter what, they will begin to see that you are not going anywhere. They don't have to amend how they feel, or who they are, for them to be supported and have someone show up for them. This is true connection, and a tremendous gift you give to them—and to you. This is trust.

Then, when there's time, open your notebook or device and transcribe their thoughts and feelings. Like how we write out our JournalSpeak instead of just thinking it, taking the time to slowly and mindfully be with our inner child's thoughts and feelings makes room for epiphany. When the sharing feels hard and painful, bathe yourself in compassion. This is a human life, flawed and shocking, complex and beautiful. Slide over on the kindergarten carpet and allow each sensation to fit. Make room for it all.

As you check in daily with your inner child, the more they will trust you, and the more they will bring to you their fears, worries, and overwhelm. Not only does this greatly decrease your reactions to triggers and the subsequent need to repress emotions, but it also directly affects your experience of pain. When your inner child is being heard more frequently, you will have more regular access to what I've described here as your higher self—the part of you that can "wear life loosely" and take each day as it comes.

As your practice deepens and evolves with consistency, throughout the day you will notice when the inner child is coming forth with a sense of despondency or overwhelm. You will also observe when they are attempting to put on the "higher self's hat" and dance as fast as they can to fix, save, and change everything. When the flustered inner child is at the helm, triggers and panic steer the ship. Yet when you show up, gently, sometimes without any obvious milestone, they'll simply stop trying to organize the pieces of your life to match their definitions of safety—which are often "safe in the unsafest way." Things that used to inflame you land softly. People with whom you share history (who were previously intolerable and insufferable) are just a nuisance now. Pain fades, and energy is made available to pursue more expansive ends.

When the higher self prevails, life feels effortless and natural. You actually become rather neutral about how things go. Can you imagine?

I have seen cosmic shifts in people (and myself) doing this work. It's emboldening to realize that we are grown and able to listen to ourselves. We don't need our parents to change, our bosses to be more sensitive, our kids not to be PITA (pain in the ass) kids. We need only presence and the willingness to witness our own grief, confusion, rage, fear, and shame with the gaze of equanimity. The bridge you build to your previously overlooked inner child is the channel that will deliver you, brick by brick.

•

Johanna's Recovery from Autoimmune Disease and Systemic Inflammation—Age 44 (Northern United States)

I spent nearly two decades of my life searching for an answer to what was making me so sick. I spent close to a hundred thousand dollars over the years on specialists, tests, and treatments that promised relief for a wide variety of symptoms with no identified common thread. From the ages of twenty to thirty-eight, I accumulated a list of twenty-three diagnoses, including IBS, cardiac arrhythmia, scoliosis, and lupus.

Some syndromes and conditions were even found accidentally during testing. After researching these incidental findings, I would develop the symptoms associated with the diagnosis. I was in tremendous pain and discomfort that was always inconsistent with measurable test results, lasted far longer than it should have, and did not respond to physical treatments. I was a medical enigma, and it was consuming my life.

Symptoms came and went in my twenties, but things really got rough when I was in my early thirties. I was in an emotionally abusive relationship and subjected daily to verbal abuse, gaslighting, and manipulation. I felt hopeless and was always afraid. My childhood trauma coexisted with this adult trauma, which I now recognize was keeping my body stuck in fight or flight.

The symptoms changed regularly, sometimes attacking all at once, rendering me bedridden and in tears for days. I had measurable systemic inflammation—my immune system was attacking itself—and I experienced so many random symptoms that it felt like my body was breaking down. I had tremors, joint pain and swelling, migraines, back pain, irregular heartbeat, chronic eye inflammation, nerve pain, gynecological issues, GI problems . . . my list of issues was a long one.

One morning while getting ready for a particularly stressful day at work, my face and ears began to swell. I was scared, and my fear exacerbated the symptoms. I tried to go about my morning, but within fifteen minutes the swelling had progressed. I was having difficulty breathing, and a sudden drop in blood pressure caused me to pass out. I was rushed to the hospital, where the ER doctor told me I had experienced anaphylactic shock and was treated with epinephrine. He was baffled to learn that I was not allergic to anything. Further testing confirmed this: I did not have any allergies, let alone one severe enough to cause anaphylaxis.

This experience added another diagnosis to my list: idiopathic anaphylaxis. In my opinion, this is the wildest (and scariest) diagnosis that turned out to be TMS! Yes, the brain really is that powerful.

As many folks do, I spent ages on the Western medicine path, searching for a common thread. I was desperate for someone to tell me that I wasn't crazy. I yearned to hear that everything could be explained by a single syndrome or disease that had yet to be found. Years after getting out of that abusive relationship, and despite being married to the most loving, supportive wife I could ever hope for, I was still in pain every day. I became more and more desperate for a unifying diagnosis that could explain everything *so I could stop fearing "it was all in my head."* (Oh, the beautiful irony.)

Then I discovered the Mindbody approach. The relief that there could be an answer to my life's search for solutions was (I know now) enough to bring my nervous system into temporary rest and repair. Within the first twelve hours I felt a reprieve from the constant pain! This gift of a small but powerful mini miracle quickly cemented my belief in the mind/body connection.

I dedicated myself to meditation and mindset management for

months, and I made some progress. I had setbacks and many symptom imperatives, and I struggled to know exactly how to get to the deep emotions that I must've been repressing to make myself so sick. In May, I came across an ad for Nicole's first retreat at the Omega Institute. It seemed like the perfect opportunity to further this journey.

The energy of community and shared purpose at the retreat kicked my healing into high gear, and JournalSpeak was the breakthrough I needed to finally release all the pent-up feelings I'd been taught over time were "shameful" or "bad" to express. Adding a JournalSpeak practice to my established meditation routine really started to shift things. I was astounded when some very difficult truths and emotions finally came to the surface . . . and subsequently left my body. I literally felt myself physically release the tension. It was magical.

Despite my immediate belief and improvement, make no mistake—this is hard work, and healing does not happen overnight. I had decades of buried trauma and emotions creating this myriad of symptoms in my body, so I needed to accept that they would not leave until my nervous system was ready. Rewiring the brain to be free of chronic pain and symptoms takes time, patience, self-love, and dedication to a JournalSpeak/meditation practice. It also requires you to be true to yourself in ways that may feel unpleasant or shameful at first.

Another key ingredient in my recovery was inner child work. I discovered that one of the reasons I developed TMS in the first place was due to a young part inside me that never felt important. Pain and being unwell used to make me (her) feel cared for and worthy of affection.

When I arrived at Omega (before I knew about inner child work or adequately understood my TMS), I sat next to someone who had a "special" chair because she had tailbone pain. I had never in my life had tailbone pain and I shit you not, intense tailbone pain was my fiercest symptom imperative! That inner child saw someone get unique treatment and extra attention for that symptom, so she generated it. And it took her a long time to trust me enough to start letting go of that debilitating pain. This work never fails to blow my mind.

Yes, this road can be difficult, uncomfortable, painful, exhausting, and time-consuming. But when you come out on the other side and finally have the rest of your life ahead of you—a life free from chronic pain and symptoms—I promise you it will all be worth it.

It's been almost five years, and I am ecstatic to report that for the first time in decades I am free of chronic conditions of any kind. I still get symptoms sometimes, but I can quickly see how they are tied to normal anxiety or emotional events, and I do the work to send them on their way. I do my JournalSpeak often, because when I don't, my system reminds me that I still need it. I am constantly in conversation with my body—and the many parts of my psyche—to better understand the protective roles that different symptoms have played in my life. In other words, I'm still rewiring my brain. Sometimes I feel frustrated that I've been doing this for so long, but then I remember that the brain is plastic and evolves throughout our entire lives. I also remind myself how much harder life was before I discovered JournalSpeak, and I shift my perspective from annoyance to gratitude. Life doesn't happen to me, it happens for me. I would choose this work any day over the agony and symptoms that kept me from living with ease.

Five years ago, I felt like I was slowly dying. Today I wholeheartedly believe that my body is healthy and capable of all it needs to be well. My quality of life has improved beyond words—physically, mentally, emotionally, and spiritually. I continue to do my best to meet myself exactly where I am on any given day, and I practice patience and kindness for myself, as Nicole so beautifully preaches.

I no longer consider my twenty-three diagnoses to be a part of me. I no longer consider them at all! Instead, I've finally found the unifying conclusion I was searching for all along—TMS—and I could not be more appreciative that the cure is within me, right at my fingertips. If you're reading this, chances are the cure is at your fingertips, too.

So take the plunge. Believe in yourself. Do this work. It is magic . . . and it will lead you home.

CHAPTER 14

TAKE BACK YOUR POWER

At the heart of this work is the idea that we need to unlearn to relearn—burn it down to build it up. We each hold the key to the jails in which we sit, and it's time to break free. Life is a choice between what hurts and what hurts worse, and you are reading this because you've realized you have a choice. The struggles that have kept you stuck are a natural reflex based on the human desire to grasp for a solution that will never materialize. As we've learned together, in any given situation there is one side of the argument and the opposing side. Believing that there is a third option—the one you prefer existed with no attendant struggle or compromise— is the delusion that keeps you stagnant and sick. Most conflict can be distilled into the following:

Option 1: Do what you are doing now.

Option 2: Do something differently.

We who have suffered in pain have tried many, many methods of recovery. Often we feel as if we've tried "everything." The ineffective treatments, procedures, meds, alternative and holistic interventions, and surgeries have taken a toll. The radical shift I am suggesting is to stop asking someone else to save you, and to understand that you have the power to save yourself.

You have arrived at this moment in your life, and endured the intense pain/anxiety/symptoms/syndromes you have, for a worthwhile reason. As the brilliant philosopher Joseph Campbell once said, "Opportunities to find deeper powers within ourselves come when life seems most challenging." You are about to discover within you the ability to heal and improve your life exponentially. You have the capability to free yourself from chronic pain, and you are ready to explore this next level of your personal evolution.

Console yourself. Your suffering has had purpose, and your struggle has not been wasted. In fact, you'll come to understand that your pain has been a gift you just didn't know how to unwrap. I've never taken seriously the word *miracle* because it's always sounded trite to me. It conjures the idea that you can't have a personal hand in your healing—that salvation must come from elsewhere, bestowed on some but not all of us. What I have found is that not only do we have a hand in our healing, but it is—at least in the case of chronic pain and anxiety—*almost entirely in our hands.* I watch people change their lives every day. It is a joy and a privilege to be part of this movement, and there is room for you in its ranks. Open yourself to the possibility that the best of your life not only is yet to come but can begin anytime you choose. New possibilities always begin with "Yes."

THIS IS YOUR LIFE

Whether you believe that our souls pass through here many times or it's one and done, this is the life where you get to be distinctly you—your hopes and dreams, your joys and sorrows, your children and families, your strengths, your talents, your challenges. This is the only one you're going to experience *just like this.* It is precious, and it matters. You are significant beyond explanation. You are unique in the world and your work here is important, no matter what it is. Whether you're managing people in a large corporation, working one-on-one in a small office, loving little people into adults, making art and exposing us all to the joys of creativity, fixing things that can't be fixed without the skills you have, or anything else—you are valued and important. We need you.

I often think about the ways this work can change the world. How many climate scientists, cancer researchers, firefighters and police officers, skyscraper builders, caring and nurturing parents, technology innovators, and other creators are at home, in bed, sidelined with chronic conditions? Awareness is the first step to changing anything. Let's stay wide awake. Let's be part of the solution in the lives of others. Let's be the truth warriors who alert those who are suffering that they have a choice.

I am here to persuade you to get uncomfortable because the road to different *is* uncomfortable. I am here to quiet your skepticism so you can speak boldly and bravely to the voice of resistance when it whispers in your ear. I want you to expect it, so it doesn't sideline you. This will allow you to do the work with belief and patience and kindness for yourself. I know you don't choose the jail you've inadvertently built around you, and I know you didn't plan for it. We all create confines around ourselves, fortified by our fear of change. There is no shame in this—it's healthy to build walls to protect yourself when you sincerely believe you're unsafe!

I am here to tell you, however, that you are indeed safer than you could possibly know. Not only is your current pain not inherently dangerous, but when you arm yourself with this knowledge and the tools to put it into action, you are protected from future illness in ways that only time will reveal. That is, if you accept this invitation I lovingly extend.

The road won't be without its bumps, which is why you need to stay conscious. Don't forget how crucial it is for you to do the work necessary to regulate your nervous system. I've had clients who'd previously allowed every new symptom to incite panic that something was physically wrong with them, even after scores of clean test results. Yet when finally they surrendered and settled into the peace of acceptance, they began to appreciate that the only way out is through. They did the work to improve their health substantially, and now they beam with the desire that you do the same.

You belong here. You are right where you need to be. You are not excluded, no matter who you are, what happened to you, where you've been, how much you've already tried, how much this runs in your family, or how many MRIs and X-rays say that you are broken. I promise you, if you do the work as I instruct with the mindset and compassion I've shared within these pages, you can be well. You can be symptom-free.

Take comfort in the amazing stories that people have offered here to inspire you. These accounts are only a tiny sampling of leagues who have healed, and I promise in some way they all look like you. Take comfort in the life-changing work of Dr. John Sarno, who brilliantly and boldly posited that much of human suffering cannot be cured through altering the physical body. Millions have thrived as a result. Take comfort in my three children, raised in this soil, who—with the correct mindset and lack of catastrophizing about their physical issues—have JournalSpoken their way out of back pain, plantar fasciitis, tendinitis, IBS, cyclical vomiting, eczema, hives, and headaches. Take comfort in the fact that you can now offer this to *your* children, who will learn and change as they observe you and follow your example. They will never become the people we were for so long—disempowered, surrendering our agency to pills, doctors, and treatments that never promised to cure our pain.

I am for you, I am with you, and I am like you. I remember my darkest days. I remember yelling in my babies' faces when I changed their diapers because my back hurt so badly I couldn't function. I remember crying myself to sleep because I thought I would never be able to travel or live a full life. I remember being hunched over with stomach pain and migraine headaches before I knew not to be afraid.

Even in these moments, I persevered. I knew from Dr. Sarno that my body would release the symptoms when my nervous system understood that I was safe. I moved through the work, and I learned as I went. I allowed my body to be my proof. I taught it to others; I lived it out loud. At age fifty-two, I stand before you, and there is nothing I can't do. My MRI remains the same. My spondylolisthesis is as shocking and disturbing on paper as it's ever been, and it was never the reason for my pain.

If I am anything at all, let me be an inspiration. If my podcast and teachings are anything at all, let them be the lifeblood in your veins as you navigate your inner world. When you are tired, rest. When your resistance wins temporarily, surrender and take a break for a day or two. But don't give up. Hold yourself in the greatest cradle of self-compassion and love. You are good, you are deserving, and you can do this. Existing in confusion, darkness, and pain is no longer the life for you. I won't have it.

As you begin to live and embody this work, I have one favor to ask of you: Please share what you have learned. From the moment I decided to teach this tool to others and venture down this windy path, I knew one thing for sure—transforming our society would never be a "top-down" endeavor. This movement would occur from the bottom up. Its momentum would build through the contribution of each individual who recognized a profound shift in their own quality of life and was called to rouse another. I envisioned these one-to-one acts of kindness growing into hundreds, thousands, and eventually millions, at which point these tools would be available to anyone who chose to be free. So if this book meant something to you, if you are better off for having read it, please gift it to someone else.

More than another volume on theory and practice, this book is meant to ignite a movement. Think of yourself as part of a humanity revolution that empowers each one of us to take back our power and "break awake," as I like to say. To break free of fear and confusion, of the emotional and physical pain that once enveloped us, so that we might wake up to the limitless possibilities that have been there all along.

It is my humblest privilege to be here with you. Take a deep breath, and let it out slowly. Your moment is here. You're ready to start living boldly and bravely with presence and resolve. You can be uncomfortable, take risks, draw boundaries, speak your truth. The former limitations of your life will soon be fodder for bittersweet stories of gratitude and wisdom. What seemed impossible is possible. What seemed inaccessible is right here, waiting to be claimed.

The gift is your life. Open it with purpose. I can't wait to see what you can do.

●

Nicole's Recovery from Pretty Much Everything—Ages 19–52 (Los Angeles, California)

I was a high-spirited child full of enthusiasm, passion, curiosity, daring, and confidence. This may sound like a great recipe for a fabulous person, but a lot of people didn't think so. My teachers said I talked too much, my friends' parents thought I was too disruptive, and my father's favorite expression when addressing me was, "Quiet down."

I was told I was careless, and I'm sure I was. I rushed through tasks and assignments wanting to be done. I moved eagerly through the world like a bull in a china shop. I raised my hand for *everything*. I cringily remember my third-grade teacher who used to survey the room and ask, "Does anyone have anything to add . . . anyone other than Nicole?" It wasn't said kindly. I was a bit too big and bold for many people's tastes. In the seventies (and also now, to some extent) children who were convenient were valued. I was not.

In tandem with this animated nature, I was a keen observer. Being raised by an unpredictable and (at times) explosive father made my organic vigilance even more pointed. I paid close attention to the way people responded to me, to their stress and annoyance, and to other kids who seemed so easily controlled. I made a judgment about myself early on that I still, at times, struggle to subdue:

I am bad. I am not the way I "should" be. I am too much. I am a disappointment.

Now, let's not play the pity violin for me quite yet. Many, many people did not find me to be any of these things. I had teachers who celebrated me. My mother regularly told me I was "Just perfect as you are!" and I had many friends who not only validated my personality but shared the same traits themselves. In retrospect, however, I know it was this dichotomy that generated much of my TMS. As we've discussed, human beings struggle with conflict more than they do anything else. When we feel strongly one way or another, we're generally able to find emotional regulation. It's when conflictual thoughts and feelings enter the picture that we experience the greatest need to repress.

None of what I'm describing to you here was conscious to me as a child. But when I look in the rearview mirror with the abundant skills I've collected over the years, I know that the divergence was banking a ton of shame. I couldn't stifle my nature and I was fairly aware that it was less than ideal. Then again, people liked me! I could be myself in lots of situations. These two energies raged an inner battle that colored the experience of my schooling, my social interactions, and my personal and familial relationships.

I had crippling insomnia as early as second grade. I would watch the clock flip from hour to hour all night, my mind spinning with panic and perseveration, fearful of what the next day would bring with no sleep. I was chronically constipated, leading to embarrassing and frightening bleeding when I could finally go. I was acutely anxious, which I had no word for at the time. This manifested as trouble swallowing and excruciating stomachaches that never seemed connected to anything I ate. I had eczema all over my body, which required special lotions and treatments through my teens. I had chronic strep throat. And, as I imagine you've gleaned by now, I had back pain. It ranged from mild and achy in my younger years to more severe as I grew, and well . . . you know the story.

My journey, however, goes far beyond the tale you've heard a hundred times if you've followed my work. It spans an adulthood of migraines, hives, chronic respiratory and other viruses, hip pain, wrist pain, elbow pain, neuropathy, bladder issues, and countless other brief encounters with many of the diagnoses you've shared with me over the years. I say this because it's essential you embrace TMS as a normal way we feel things. I am human, and (sometimes annoyingly) there is no being "better" or "done" with that. Any sensation I ever experience is temporary. Sometimes we feel things in our hearts, sometimes we feel things in our bodies, and they are interchangeable. In my decades of helping all manner of people walk this path, I have come to not only accept this but to celebrate it.

TMS has cracked me open, again and again. It's forced me to stop in my tracks and pay attention to the things that need to be felt in my heart and mind. It's commanded that I grow. No one is more grateful for their pain than I am. It's revealed possibilities that I'd never considered, as the epiphanies generated in doing the work have taught me what I really think and feel. And oh my *God*—the privilege it's afforded me to help *you*. To know you, and see you, and feel your humanity. I am floored by my good luck, yet it's all come in packages one might've labeled as "suffering." We have the power to rewrite this narrative. What if suffering is grace? What if, as the mystic poet Rumi wrote, "the wound is the place where the light enters you"?

This doesn't mean I don't take new symptoms seriously. When I got burning mouth syndrome a few years ago, I busted through my doctor's door, sure I was dying. "I think I taste pennies!" I blurted out. "Am I having a stroke?"

She took my vitals and did bloodwork, but the most valuable thing she said was, rather offhandedly, "You know, I have another patient with these symptoms. She's been struggling for over a year and even went to the Mayo Clinic to get herself checked out. They think it has something to do with *stress*!" Needless to say, that was all I needed to hear. I all but danced out the door with my normal bloodwork and vitals and proceeded home to do the work with "burning mouth" as my focus. The symptoms abated soon enough.

The most important transformation I can share with you is that no matter the way TMS has presented itself (and continues to do from time to time), I am never afraid. I get checked out if I need to, and I take medication or have procedures as appropriate. But as soon as I feel comfortable that the symptom isn't structural or infectious in nature, I just relax and do the work. Nothing chronic has owned me for years and years, and on most days I feel fantastic. This is the definition of peace.

There will never be a day when everything in the world aligns exactly the way I want or "need" it to. Peace means I am centered and confident, even when it doesn't. Peace means that I can stand in the middle of my proverbial chaos—in mind, body, family, situation—and do what's necessary to take care of myself. Regardless of the moment's discomfort, I know that when my nervous system is ready to regulate, I will be pain-free. This is where I live.

My children are being raised with this work as their guiding force. My oldest is an artist studying in a rigorous college program. Sometimes when her back hurts or her eczema flares, she calls me and says, "*Ugh!* I have to get to my JournalSpeak!" She may experience resistance—it's human nature—but she knows what to do to help herself. The same is true of my son with his anxiety and my youngest daughter, a dancer, who gets the aches and pains associated with her passion without ever allowing them to become chronic. She laments when she sees dear friends sitting out with persistent "injuries," and she does her best to open them to this work. As I continue down the path of bringing these practices to the global community, I look forward to helping younger people understand the genius of TMS recovery. There is so much needless suffering that must be transmuted.

The doctors who diagnosed me when I was nineteen were not incompetent, ill-intentioned, or irresponsible. They were doing the best they could with the knowledge they had at the time. Having said that, they were dead wrong. I run, I travel, I carried three babies to term without incident, and I am the first to grab my ridiculously overpacked suitcase and toss it into the trunk. I am healthy. I am strong. And I am free.

It's your turn. Don't be afraid. Your freedom is worth the journey, whatever challenges it brings. You will never again be alone in your pain. We are an army of warriors who march beside you. We surround you with love, we remind you that you have power, and we celebrate you as you awaken. This is your life. Now go, and take it back.

APPENDIX

FREQUENTLY ASKED QUESTIONS (FAQ)

HOW DO I FIND ALL OF NICOLE'S RESOURCES AND GUIDANCE?

Go to my website www.nicolesachs.com. It is continually updated with all of our new offerings and opportunities to learn with me (and team) LIVE and virtually. It also has a Podcast page, where you can search for any specific symptom or topic.

WHAT ARE THE THREE FACETS OF NICOLE'S WORK?

· Believe
· Do the work
· Practice patience and kindness for yourself (*self-compassion* is a verb!)

IS IT NORMAL FOR MY SYMPTOMS TO GET WORSE/ CHANGE/MOVE AROUND WHEN I FIRST START JOURNALSPEAK?

Yes, yes, and yes. JournalSpeak stirs up difficult emotions that you've been suppressing for a long time. There is often a physical backlash as your nervous system desperately tries to keep you "safe" from the feelings that are rising. It's very common for symptoms to get worse initially, for new symptoms to appear, and for symptoms to move around your body—for example, from one hip to the other, from your lower back to your upper back, or even to your stomach or head. This is the symptom imperative, as Dr. Sarno coined it, and although it feels like a backslide, it's actually good news! You've got the symptoms on the run, and they are moving around to move out of your body. Keep telling yourself that you're safe, that this isn't a physical problem (it has an emotional genesis, even though it is physically very real), and take these things as proof that something is shifting, which means it's working!

HOW LONG WILL IT TAKE ME TO HEAL?

This is what everyone wants to know, but there is no one-size-fits-all answer. A rare few recover almost instantly on discovering the Mindbody connection, but they aren't the majority. Even these people must do the deeper work to protect themselves from symptom imperatives down the road. Most people experience a more gradual recovery that can take weeks, months, or even longer. Also, recovery is not a straight line. There will be peaks and troughs along the way, so don't be disheartened if you have bad days even when things have started to improve.

WHAT IF I RELAPSE?

As stated previously, ups and downs are to be expected during recovery. Occasional relapses or symptom flares are a normal part of the process. If and when this happens, don't panic. This fuels them with fear. Try to practice acceptance and patience/kindness for yourself, and keep JournalSpeaking and using meditation.

WHAT CAN I DO TO SOOTHE AND CALM MY NERVOUS SYSTEM?

Use meditation, acceptance, and breathing exercises, and seek support from my private Facebook group (JournalSpeak with Nicole Sachs, LCSW) and Instagram community (@nicolesachslcsw) to know you're not alone. Listening to my podcast can open the door to community and solace as well. Search for it wherever you get your podcasts—*The Cure for Chronic Pain* with Nicole Sachs, LCSW. There are so many resources available and new ones being offered all the time at my website: www.nicolesachs.com.

IS IT NORMAL TO EXPERIENCE ANXIETY AND/OR DEPRESSION WHEN PHYSICAL SYMPTOMS START TO IMPROVE?

Yes, this is just part of the symptom imperative. One person's back pain is another person's anxiety. Just keep swimming.

DOES IT MATTER IF I JOURNAL ABOUT THE SAME THINGS OVER AND OVER?

No! This is great. Feel it all until you have the deep peace of being okay with it.

WON'T IT MAKE ME FEEL WORSE IF I DWELL ON NEGATIVE THINGS?

No. This is one of the biggest misconceptions of TMS work. If you stay the course and allow yourself to be open to the stream of life it invites, you will feel freer than ever before.

CAN I STILL GET PHYSICAL THERAPY/GET MASSAGES/SEE A CHIROPRACTOR?

There are two main energies in the universe: love and fear. If you do things out of desperation to heal (fear), it will trigger your nervous system into fight or flight and make you worse. If you get the massage (with love) to connect with your body, then it is good for you. Physical therapy and chiropractic were not advised by Dr. Sarno, but can still be acceptable for reasons other than chronic pain recovery (strengthening the body, being in alignment). If you choose to engage in them, practice going out of love to gain support instead of "fixing yourself."

HOW DO I EXERCISE WITH PAIN?

If you can do it out of love and health, exercising through the pain will not hurt you. Don't push it—do what feels comfortable to you.

HOW DO I EXPLAIN TMS TO MY FAMILY, PARTNER, FRIENDS, AND OTHERS?

Perhaps show them my website (www.nicolesachs.com) or invite them to listen to my four-part *Healing Yourself* series on The Cure for Chronic Pain YouTube channel with you. Just remember that this is a program of attraction, not promotion. Your people may question whether an emotional exercise can cure a physical condition, and that's their prerogative. Allow friends and loved ones to have their feelings, and lead with quiet confidence. As you get better, your body becomes your proof—and theirs.

If you are a practitioner, clinician, teacher, coach, or community leader who wants real, solid guidance in communicating this to others, go to www.sarnosachs.com to learn about the training we created with Christina Sarno Horner. It gives you the comprehensive toolkit necessary to carry this message and live it most robustly yourself.

ACKNOWLEDGMENTS

There was never a time I would've given up, but there was a time I was tired. For many years I largely went it alone. I wrote my first self-published book, created TCFCP website and YouTube channel, launched the podcast, and showed up every day on Instagram. I carried this message as best I could, hoping that the collective consciousness would shift just enough to allow me a greater voice.

Lisa Eisenpresser, you walked into my world with your dazzling smile, brilliant mind, years of entrepreneurial wisdom, and immediate knowing that these teachings were meant to, as you say, "blanket the planet" and save lives. Thank you. Thank you for your uncanny ability to learn and understand the most nuanced theories and turn around and explain them with clarity and confidence. Thank you for your mindful and steady awareness of what is most important, and your unapologetic ability to communicate it. Thank you for being a true partner in every sense of the word, and undoubtedly making me, this message, our communities, and our lives fuller, richer, and better. And finally, thank you for doing this work like a warrior to banish your own migraines and allow your body to be your proof. I never feel alone anymore. When one day soon, the ground swells with people from all over the world taking back their health, power, joy, and presence, it will unquestionably be because of you and all you've brought to this movement. I love you.

Thank you to Joy Tutela, my incomparable literary agent, who saw a wink from the universe in the name of my mentor Dr. John Sarno and said, "Let's do this!" Your belief in me and this work and your steadfast partnership in all things publishing have been invaluable. I'm honored to walk beside you. Thank you also to Kayt Sukel for being my very first reader and offering such helpful insights and feedback with a "newcomer's" brain.

Thank you, Dr. Sarno. Your bravery and tenacity to create and teach these theories for years against all odds will not be forgotten. Thank you also to Christina Sarno Horner for being a partner in carrying these transformative practices to clinicians, therapists, and all those looking to enhance their communities with this work. May the *Sarno x Sachs Solution* further our cause exponentially. Thank you to Veronica Domingo and all of the amazing people at the Omega Institute for giving us a home each summer to guide people in taking their healing to the next level.

Thank you to Nina Shield, Hannah Steigmeyer, and the team at Penguin Random House for seeing the necessity and timeliness of this book, and giving it the perfect home in which to grow and prepare for its trip around the world. I can't wait to see what it will do under your care. Thank you to Art Streiber and the most professional and kick-ass photography crew. You captured the exact me I'm proud to share with the world.

Thank you to my adoring Mama, a mother any daughter would pick should she have the chance. Your mantra, which rings in my mind daily, "Why not you?!" has propelled me through every hesitation, fear of rejection, impatience, and longing. There has never been a time that I felt you were not only on my side, but my impassioned champion. If everyone had a mother like you, I can't imagine there would be so much pain in the world. Thank you for giving me the confidence to jump back into the fray every time I was pushed aside. You are the genesis of everything I'm able to give others.

Thank you to my beautiful babies, who might never have been had I bent to the fear and meaning attached to that dark diagnosis at age nineteen. Isabella, Oliver, and Charlotte, you are my greatest achievements, if I can call you mine. You are yours, and there is nothing more joyful than watching each of you meet every complex challenge with the values and grit that I hope to have modeled. You are introspective, thoughtful, loving, and generous people, and there is nothing for which I feel more gratitude than the fact you walk the earth. You've taught me how to love fiercely, and your existence makes it possible for me to shine my light on the world.

Thank you to my wonderful modern family. May we teach the world that there are many ways to define kin. Kate and Phoebe, how did I get so lucky to have such magnificent bonus babies? It must be because we've walked the earth together for many lifetimes. I love you as much as if I'd carried you myself, and it's sometimes hard to believe I didn't, with our freakishly aligned tastes and personalities. I love you both so much. Stella and Dawn, you broke me in as a stepmom and showed me that raising five kids won't (necessarily) kill you. I love you always.

Special thanks to Kate for taking on the role of Teen Ambassador and showing me how profoundly capable a teenager is of learning and living this work. Having not been raised in this soil, your embodiment of this message gives me tremendous hope that we will succeed in bringing healing to younger and younger people.

David, my forever parenting partner, thank you for always having my back when it comes to these angelic children. You call this a happy family?! Martha, Margaret, Dan, Chris, Sarah, and Jenny, thank you for making me feel held, supported, and loved. I am so lucky to be by Lisa's side and to have inherited such a wonderful "framily." Special thanks to the group chat (whose name will remain unspoken) for coming up with the title *Mind Your Body*.

Thank you to my incredible circle of friends and colleagues who share this journey with me. To my best friend, Danielle Furst, your music has been the soundtrack for Omega, the podcast, and many of my most joyful moments. I cherish our sisterhood and everything it fuels. Robin Ruzan, the deep dive on Google that led you to me started everything. Thank you for being a partner on this quest and so many others. Shoshana Bean, you embraced this work and jumped in with four paws. Your gorgeous, powerful voice is a living testament to its efficacy. Jessica Caiola-Rich, PhD, you healed yourself and now you bring that healing to others. Grateful for you, Theresa, and all you've both brought to my life. Michael Porter Jr., your willingness to look outside of the box and find your way to healing after three back surgeries will change the lives of men and athletes worldwide.

Lisa Schlosberg and Caroline Dewey, you will always be my OG Team, and I thank you profoundly for our years of working and playing together. I look forward to all you'll add to the wellness space that will undoubtedly help so many. Gigi Cockell, you bring the scientific expertise so sorely needed where confusion can obscure belief. Thank you for your recovery, your infectious energy, and your essential contributions to our communities. Ali, Michelle, Ash, and the team at Soul Camp Creative, your partnership in conceiving and building BreakAwake has provided the solid foundation on which all will be built.

Thank you to my admins who've donated so generously of their time and energy to moderate the JournalSpeak FB community over the years: Angie, Claire, Deb, Enda, Erika, Justine, Kat, Kai, Kira, Kristen, Melanie, Melissa, Monica, Nyle, Phil, Preetha, Scarlett— you are invaluable in your kindness, generosity, and wisdom. Thank you for giving of yourself to such a worthy cause.

To my dad, your influence on my values, work ethic, confidence, and character is still going strong twenty-five years after you left us. I deeply honor and value our work together in this life. Uncle Charlie, I'm so grateful to have your love, support, and living connection to my father and our complex family history.

Thank you, Bludog. I love you, and I know you're here.

Finally, my heartfelt thanks to the beautiful souls who shared their personal stories within these pages, our BreakAwake Membership Community, and every one of you who didn't give up when you were handed a diagnosis without a cure, years of suffering without a solution, and many moments of darkness where light wasn't readily available. You are my beacon. You are the reason I never considered laying down my pen.

With love,
Nicole

FURTHER READING:
BOOKS AND SCIENTIFIC STUDIES

ON TENSION MYONEURAL SYNDROME (TMS)

Coen, S. J., and J. E. Sarno. "Psychosomatic avoidance of conflict in back pain." *Journal of the American Academy of Psychoanalysis* 17, no. 3 (1989): 359–376.

Sarno, John E., MD. *The Divided Mind: The Epidemic of Mindbody Disorders.* New York: HarperCollins, 2007.

———. *Healing Back Pain: The Mind-Body Connection.* New York: Warner Books, 1991.

———. *Mind over Back Pain: A Radically New Approach to the Diagnosis and Treatment of Back Pain.* New York: Brilliance, 1982.

———. *The Mindbody Prescription: Healing the Body, Healing the Pain.* New York: Warner Books, 1998.

ON THE NEUROBIOLOGY OF PAIN

Baller, Erica B., and David A. Ross. "Your system has been hijacked: The neurobiology of chronic pain." *Biological Psychiatry* 82, no. 8 (2017): e61–e63.

Bushnell, M. Catherine, Marta Ceko, and Lucie A. Low. "Cognitive and emotional control of pain and its disruption in chronic pain." *Nature Reviews Neuroscience* 14, no. 7 (2013): 502–511.

De Ridder, Dirk, Divya Adhia, and Sven Vanneste. "The anatomy of pain and suffering in the brain and its clinical implications." *Neuroscience and Biobehavioral Reviews* 130 (2021): 125–146.

Fenton, Bradford W., Elim Shih, and Jessica Zolton. "The neurobiology of pain perception in normal and persistent pain." *Pain Management* 5, no. 4 (2015): 297–317.

Garland, Eric. "Pain processing in the human nervous system: A selective review of nociceptive and biobehavioral pathways." *Primary Care* 39, no. 3 (2012): 561–571.

Know, Mikwang, Murat Altin, Hector Duenas, and Levent Alev. "The role of descending inhibitory pathways on chronic pain modulation and clinical implications." *Pain Practice* 14, no. 7 (2014): 656–667.

Kross, Ethan, Marc G. Berman, Walter Mischel, Edward E. Smith, and Tor D. Wager. "Social rejection shares somatosensory representations with physical pain." *PNAS* 108, no. 15 (2011): 6270–6275.

Ossipov, Michael H., Kozo Morimura, and Frank Porreca, "Descending pain modulation and chronicification." *Current Opinion on Supportive and Palliative Care* 8, no. 2 (2014): 143–151.

Stegemann, Alina, Sheng Liu, Oscar Andres Retana Romero, Manfred Josef Oswald, Yechao Han, Carlo Antonio Berretta, Zheng Gan, Linette Liqi Tan, William Wisden, Johannes Graff, and Rohini Kuner. "Prefrontal engrams of long-term fear memory perpetuate pain perception." *Nature Neuroscience* 26 (2023): 820–829.

ON THE BIOPSYCHOSOCIAL MODEL OF CHRONIC PAIN AND PHYSICAL ILLNESS

Atlas, Lauren Y., and Mustafa al'Absi. "The neuroscience of pain: Biobehavioral, developmental, and psychosocial mechanisms relevant to intervention targets." *Psychosomatic Medicine* 80, no. 9 (2018): 788–790.

Farrell, Scott F., Pik-Fang Kho, Mischa Lundberg, Adrian I. Campos, Miguel E. Renteria, Rutger M. J. de Zoete, Michele Sterling, Trung Thanh Ngo, and Gabriel Cuellar-Partida. "A shared genetic signature for common chronic pain conditions and its impact on biopsychosocial traits." *Journal of Pain* 24, no. 3 (2023): 369–386.

Gatchel, Robert J., Yuan Bo Peng, Madelon L. Peters, Perry N. Fuchs, and Dennis C. Turk. "The biopsychosocial approach to chronic pain: Scientific advances and future directions." *Psychological Bulletin* 133, no. 4 (2007): 581–624.

Meints, S. M., and R. R. Edwards. "Evaluating psychosocial contributions to chronic pain outcomes." *Progress in Neuro-Psychopharmacology and Biological Psychiatry* 87, Part B (2018): 168–182.

Pace-Schott, Edward F., Marlissa C. Amole, Tatjana Aue, Michela Balconi, Lauren M. Bylsma, Hugo Critchley, Heath A. Demaree, Bruce H. Friedman, Anne Elizabeth Kotynski Gooding, Olivia Gosseries, Tanja Jovanovic, Lauren A. J. Kirby, Kasa Kozlowska, Steven Laureys, Leroy Lowe, Kelsey Magee, Marie-France Marin, Amanda R. Merner, Jennifer L. Robinson, Robert C. Smith, Derek P. Spangler, Mark Van Overveld, and Michael B. VanElzakker. "Physiological feelings." *Neuroscience and Biobehavioral Reviews* 103 (2019): 267–304.

Purdy, Jana. "Chronic physical illness: A psychophysiological approach for chronic physical illness." *Yale Journal of Biology and Medicine* 86, no. 1 (2013): 15–28.

Tanguay-Sabourin, Christophe, Matt Fillingim, Gianluca V. Guglietti, Azin Zare, Marc Parisien, Jax Norman, Hilary Sweatman, Ronrick Da-ano, Eveliina Heikkala, PREVENT-AD Research Group, Jordi Perez, Jaro Karppinen, Sylvia Villeneuve, Scott J. Thompson, Marc O. Martel, Mathieu Roy, Luda Diatchenko, and Etienne Vachon-Presseau. "A prognostic risk score for development and spread of chronic pain." *Nature Medicine* 29 (2023): 1821–1831.

ON THE IMPACT OF EMOTIONAL PROCESSING ON CHRONIC CONDITIONS

Ashar, Yoni K., Alan Gordon, and Howard Schubiner. "Effect of pain reprocessing therapy vs. placebo and usual care for patients with chronic back pain: A randomized clinical trial." *JAMA Psychiatry* 79, no. 1 (2021): 13–23, doi:10.1001/jamapsychiatry.2021.2669.

Donnino, Michael W., Patricia Howard, Shivani Mehta, Jeremy Silverman, Maria J. Cabrera, Jolin B. Yamin, Lakshman Balaji, Katherine M. Berg, Stanley Heydrick, Robert Edwards, and Anne V. Grossestreuer. "Psychophysiologic symptom relief therapy for post-acute sequelae of COVID-19: A non-randomized interventional study." *Mayo Clinic Proceedings: Innovations, Quality & Outcomes* 7, no. 4 (2023): 337–348.

Donnino, Michael W., Garrett S. Thompson, Shivani Mehta, Myrella Paschali, Patricia Howard, Sofie B. Antonsen, Lakshman Balaji, Suzanne M. Bertisch, Robert Edwards, Long H. Ngo, and Anne V. Grossestreuer. "Psychophysiologic symptom relief therapy for chronic back pain: A pilot randomized controlled trial." *Pain Reports* 6, no. 3 (2021): doi:10.1097/PR9.0000000000000959.

McCracken, Lance, Lin Yu, and Kevin E. Vowles. "New generation psychological treatments in chronic pain." *British Medical Journal* 376 (2022): e057212.

Quartana, P. J., and J. W. Burns. "Painful consequences of anger suppression." *Emotion* 7, no. 2 (2007): 400–414.

Tankha, Hallie, Mark A. Lumley, Alan Gordon, Howard Schubiner, Christie Uipi, James Harris, Tor D. Wager, and Yoni K. Ashar. "'I don't have chronic back pain anymore': Patient experiences in pain reprocessing therapy for chronic back pain." *Journal of Pain* 24, no. 9 (2023): 1582–1593.

Thakur, E. R., H. J. Holmes, N. A. Lockhart, J. N. Carty, M. S. Ziadni, H. K. Doherty, J. M. Lacker, H. Schubiner, and M. A. Lumley. "Emotional awareness and expression training improves irritable bowel syndrome: A randomized controlled trial." *Neurogastroenterology and Motility* 29, no. 12 (2017): e13143.

ON THE NEUROSCIENCE OF MEDITATION

Kral, Tammi R. A., Brianna S. Schuyler, Jeanette A. Mumford, Melissa A. Rosenkranz, Antoine Lutz, and Richard J. Davidson. "Impact of short- and long-term mindfulness meditation training on amygdala reactivity to emotional stimuli." *Neuroimage* 181 (2018): 301–313.

Prakash, Ruchika Shaurya. "Mindfulness meditation: Impact on attentional control and emotional dysregulation." *Archives of Clinical Neuropsychology* 37, no. 7 (2021): 1283–1290.

Tang, Yi-Yuan, Britta K. Holzel, and Michael I. Posner. "The neuroscience of mindfulness meditation." *Nature Reviews Neuroscience* 16, no. 4 (2015): 213–225.

NOTES

EPIGRAPH

vii **Mental pain is less dramatic:** C. S. Lewis, *The Problem of Pain* (New York: Macmillan, 1944).

AUTHOR'S NOTE

xvii **Around the globe:** Daniel S. Goldberg and Summer J McGee, "Pain as a global public health priority," *BMC Public Health* 11 (2011): 770; Cother Hajat and Emma Stein, "The global burden of multiple chronic conditions: A narrative review," *Preventive Medicine Reports* 12 (2018): 284–293.

CHAPTER 1: MINDBODY MEDICINE EXPLAINED

3 **I finally stopped avoiding fires:** Glennon Doyle, *Untamed* (New York: Dial Press, 2020).

6 **He referred to this condition:** John E. Sarno, MD, *Mind over Back Pain: A Radically New Approach to the Diagnosis and Treatment of Back Pain* (New York: Brilliance, 1982).

7 **After reading *Healing Back Pain*:** John E. Sarno, MD, *Healing Back Pain: The Mind-Body Connection* (New York: Warner Books, 1991).

8 **Despite the fact that scientific studies:** Marie Hoeger Bement, Andy Weyer, Manda Keller, April L. Harkins, and Sandra K. Hunter. "Anxiety and stress can predict pain perception following a cognitive stress," *Physiology and Behavior* 101, no. 1 (2010): 87–92.

8 **Instead, they refer to psychophysiological symptoms:** M. Luisa Figueira and Silvia Ouakinin, "From psychosomatic to psychological

medicine: What's the future?," *Current Opinions in Psychiatry* 21, no. 4 (2008): 412–416, https://doi.org/10.1097/YCO.0b013e328300c731.

9 **This diversion process:** Kasia Kozlowska, Peter Walker, Loyola McLean, and Pascal Carrive, "Fear and the defense cascade: Clinical implications and management," *Harvard Review of Psychiatry* 23, no. 4 (2015): 263–287.

9 **These chemicals raise both your respiratory and heart rates:** Goran Simic, Mladenka Tkalcic, Vana Vukic, Damir Mulc, Ena Spanic, Marina Sagud, Francisco E. Olucha-Bordonau, Mario Vuksic, and Patrick R. Hof, "Understanding emotions: Origins and roles of the amygdala," *Biomolecules* 11, no. 6 (2021): 823.

9 **Whether your amygdala directs you:** Bruce S. McEwan, PhD, "The brain on stress: Toward an integrative approach to brain, body, and behavior," *Perspectives in Psychological Science* 8, no. 6 (2013): 673–675.

12 **Once you become totally enmeshed:** John E. Sarno, MD, *Healing Back Pain: The Mind-Body Connection* (New York: Warner Books, 1991).

16 **Many tests, scans, probes:** N. Boos, Rico Rieder, Volker Schade, K. Spratt, N. Semmer, and M. Aebi, "The diagnostic accuracy of magnetic resonance imaging, work perception, and psychosocial factors in identifying symptomatic disc herniations," *Spine* 20 (1995): 2613–2625; D. G. Borenstein, J. W. O'Mara Jr., W. C. Lauerman, A. Jacobson, C. Platenberg, D. Schellinger, and S. W. Wiesel, "The value of magnetic resonance imaging of the lumbar spine to predict low-back pain in asymptomatic subjects: A seven-year follow-up study," *Journal of Bone and Joint Surgery* 83, no. 9 (2001): 1306–1311; Martin Englund, Ali Guermazi, Daniel Gale, David J. Hunter, Piran Aliabadi, Margaret Clancy, and David T. Felson, "Incidental meniscal findings on knee MRI in middle-aged and elder persons," *New England Journal of Medicine* 359, no. 11 (2008): 1108–1115.

16 **But when researchers at the Mayo Clinic reviewed:** W. Brinjikji, P. H. Luetmer, B. Comstock, B. W. Bresnahan, L. E. Chen, R. A. Deyo, S. Halabi, J. A. Turner, A. L. Avins, K. James, J. T. Wald, D. F. Kallmes, and J. G. Jarvik, "Systematic literature review of imaging features of spinal degeneration in asymptomatic populations,"

American Journal of Neuroradiology 36, no. 4 (April 2015): 811–816, https://doi.org/10.3174/ajnr.A4173.

CHAPTER 2: A WHOLE CHAPTER ON THE BRAIN SCIENCE

27 **The reason anyone suffers:** Eric Garland, "Pain processing in the human nervous system: A selective review of nociceptive and biobehavioral pathways," *Primary Care* 39, no. 3 (2012): 561–571.

28 **This is the spot:** Goran Simic, Mladenka Tkalcic, Vana Vukic, Damir Mulc, Ena Spanic, Marina Sagud, Francisco E. Olucha-Bordonau, Mario Vuksic, and Patrick R. Hof, "Understanding emotions: Origins and roles of the amygdala," *Biomolecules* 11, no. 6 (2021): 823.

28 **Pain is the messenger:** "'Ouch, that hurts!' The science of pain," *NIH MedlinePlus*, May 23, 2023, https://magazine.medlineplus.gov /article/ouch-that-hurts-the-science-of-pain.

28 **The amygdala, which is sometimes referred to:** James Sullivan, "Know your brain: The amygdala—unlocking your reptilian brain," *Brain World Magazine*, December 29, 2021, https://brainworld magazine.com/know-your-brain-the-amygdala-unlocking-the -reptilian-brain/.

29 **The brain not only has the capacity:** V. Tabry, T. A. Vogel, M. Lussier, P. Brouillard, J. Buhle, P. Rainville, L. Bherer, and M. Roy, "Inter-individual predictors of pain inhibition during performance of a competing cognitive task," *Scientific Reports* 10 (2020).

30 **Take note again:** Dirk De Ridder, Divya Adhia, and Sven Vanneste, "The anatomy of pain and suffering in the brain and its clinical implications," *Neuroscience and Biobehavioral Reviews* 130 (2021): 125–146.

30 **The brain's evolution:** Alina Stegemann, Sheng Liu, Oscar Andres Retana Romero, Manfred Josef Oswald, Yechao Han, Carlo Antonio Berretta, Zheng Gan, Linette Liqi Tan, William Wisden, Johannes Graff, and Rohini Kuner, "Prefrontal engrams of long-term fear memory perpetuate pain perception," *Nature Neuroscience* 26 (2023): 820–829.

32 **The most effective protective posture:** John E. Sarno, MD, *Healing Back Pain: The Mind-Body Connection* (New York: Warner Books, 1991).

32 **Many are now advocating:** S. M. Meints and R. R. Edwards, "Evaluating psychosocial contributions to chronic pain outcomes," *Progress in Neuro-Psychopharmacology and Biological Psychiatry* 87, Part B (2018): 168–182.

33 **And as scientists are learning:** S. M. Meints and R. R. Edwards, "Evaluating psychosocial contributions to chronic pain outcomes," *Progress in Neuro-Psychopharmocology and Biological Psychiatry* 87, Part B (2018): 168–182.

33 **But what is happening in your head:** Erica B. Baller and David A. Ross, "Your system has been hijacked: The neurobiology of chronic pain," *Biological Psychiatry* 82, no. 8 (2017): e61–e63.

34 **The signals/neural pathways activated:** Ethan Kross, Marc G. Berman, Walter Mischel, Edward E. Smith, and Tor D. Wager, "Social rejection shares somatosensory representations with physical pain." *PNAS* 108, no. 15 (2011): 6270–6275.

36 **Van der Kolk shows:** Bessel van der Kolk, MD, *The Body Keeps the Score: Brain, Mind, and Body in the Healing of Trauma* (New York: Penguin Books, 2014).

36 **Maté looks at the links:** Gabor Maté, MD, *When the Body Says No: The Cost of Hidden Stress* (New York: Vermilion, 2019).

37 **These are all emotional stimuli:** Edward F. Pace-Schott, Marlissa C. Amole, Tatjana Aue, Michela Balconi, Lauren M. Bylsma, Hugo Critchley, Heath A. Demaree, Bruce H. Friedman, Anne Elizabeth Kotynski Gooding, Olivia Gosseries, Tanja Jovanovic, Lauren A. J. Kirby, Kasa Kozlowska, Steven Laureys, Leroy Lowe, Kelsey Magee, Marie-France Marin, Amanda R. Merner, Jennifer L. Robinson, Robert C. Smith, Derek P. Spangler, Mark Van Overveld, and Michael B. VanElzakker, "Physiological feelings," *Neuroscience and Biobehavioral Reviews* 103 (2019): 267–304.

37 **Many traditionally held medical tropes:** D. G. Borenstein, J. W. O'Mara Jr., W. C. Lauerman, A. Jacobson, C. Platenberg, D. Schellinger, and S. W. Wiesel, "The value of magnetic resonance imaging of the lumbar spine to predict low-back pain in asymptomatic subjects: A seven-year follow-up study," *Journal of Bone and Joint Surgery* 83, no. 9 (2001): 1306–1311.

38 **That led Donnino to conclude:** Michael W. Donnino, Garrett S. Thompson, Shivani Mehta, Myrella Paschali, Patricia Howard, Sofie B. Antonsen, Lakshman Balaji, Suzanne M. Bertisch, Robert Edwards, Long H. Ngo, and Anne V. Grossestreuer, "Psychophysiologic symptom relief therapy for chronic back pain: A pilot randomized controlled trial," *Pain Reports* 6, no. 3 (2021), doi:10.1097/PR9.0000000000000959.

38 **Once again, when Donnino:** Michael Donnino, Patricia Howard, Shivani Mehta, Jeremy Silverman, Maria J. Cabrera, Jolin B. Yamin, Lakshman Balaji, Katherine M. Berg, Stanley Heydrick, Robert Edwards, and Anne V. Grossestreuer, "Psychophysiologic symptom relief therapy for post-acute sequelae of COVID-19: A nonrandomized interventional study," *Mayo Clinic Proceedings: Innovations, Quality & Outcomes* 7, no. 4 (2023): 337–348.

39 **Researchers at Weill Cornell Medical Center:** Yoni K. Ashar, Alan Gordon, and Howard Schubiner, "Effect of pain reprocessing therapy vs. placebo and usual care for patients with chronic back pain: A randomized clinical trial," *JAMA Psychiatry* 79, no. 1 (2021): 1323, doi:10.1001/jamapsychiatry.2021.2669; Hallie Tankha, Mark A. Lumley, Alan Gordon, Howard Schubiner, Christie Uipi, James Harris, Tor D. Wager, and Yoni K. Ashar, "'I don't have chronic back pain anymore': Patient experiences in pain reprocessing therapy for chronic back pain," *Journal of Pain* 24, no. 9 (2023): 1582–1593.

39 **Another group of researchers:** E. R. Thakur, H. J. Holmes, N. A. Lockhart, J. N. Carty, M. S. Ziadni, H. K. Doherty, J. M. Lacker, H. Schubiner, and M. A. Lumley, "Emotional awareness and expression training improves irritable bowel syndrome: A randomized controlled trial," *Neurogastroenterology and Motility* 29, no. 12 (2017): e13143.

39 **Regardless of diagnosis:** P. J. Quartana and J. W. Burns. "Painful consequences of anger suppression," *Emotion* 7, no. 2 (2007): 400–414.

CHAPTER 3: MINDSET: YOUR PERCEPTION IS YOUR REALITY

45 **If you perceive yourself to be unsafe:** Anne Trafton, "How expectation influences perception," *MIT News*, July 15, 2019, https://news.mit.edu/2019/how-expectation-influences-perception-0715.

47 **In Buddhism:** Thich Nhat Hanh, *The Heart of the Buddha's Teaching: Transforming Suffering into Peace, Joy, and Liberation* (New York: Harmony Books, 1999).

CHAPTER 4: SOME QUESTIONS TO CONSIDER ABOUT YOU

63 **"Start as you mean to go on":** Tracy Hogg with Melinda Blau, *Secrets of the Baby Whisperer: How to Calm, Connect, and Communicate with Your Baby* (New York: Ballantine Books, 2001).

66 **We can move forward:** Ann M. Graybiel and Kyle S. Smith, "How the brain makes and breaks habits," *Scientific American*, June 2014.

71 **In her book *White Hot Truth*:** Danielle LaPorte, *White Hot Truth: Clarity for Keeping It Real on Your Spiritual Path—from One Seeker to Another* (Vancouver, Canada: Virtuonica, 2017).

CHAPTER 5: EXPECTATION SETTING IS EVERYTHING (OR OVERCOMING RESISTANCE)

84 **When you are in a chronically stressed state:** Emma Seppälä, "Your high-intensity feelings may be wearing you out," *Harvard Business Review*, February 2016, https://hbr.org/2016/02/your-high -intensity-feelings-may-be-tiring-you-out.

85 **The seventeenth-century Dutch philosopher:** Benedict de Spinoza, *Ethics, Demonstrated in Geometrical Order (Ethica, Ordine Geometrico Demonstrata)*, 1677.

87 **The *symptom imperative*, a term:** John E. Sarno, MD, *Healing Back Pain: The Mind-Body Connection* (New York: Warner Books, 1991).

92 **Ram Dass, the famed American spiritual leader:** Ram Dass, *Be Here Now* (New York: Harmony Books, 1978).

94 **When explaining TMS:** John E. Sarno, MD, *The Divided Mind: The Epidemic of Mindbody Disorders* (New York: HarperCollins, 2007).

CHAPTER 8: JOURNALSPEAK AND MEDITATION ARE YOUR VEHICLES TO FREEDOM

148 **Dozens of neuroscience studies:** Kayt Sukel, "Understanding the power of meditation," BrainFacts.org, April 19, 2019, https://www .brainfacts.org/thinking-sensing-and-behaving/thinking-and -awareness/2019/understanding-the-power-of-meditation-041919.

148 **Studies done by researchers:** Haiteng Jiang, Bin He, Xialoi Guo, Xu Wang, Menglin Guo, Zhuo Wang, Ting Xue, Han Li, Tianjiao Xu, Shuai Ye, Daniel Suma, Shanbao Tong, and Donghong Cui, "Brain-heart interactions underlying traditional Tibetan Buddhist meditation," *Cerebral Cortex* 30, no. 20 (2020): 439–450.

CHAPTER 9: EVOLVE YOUR JOURNALSPEAK

167 **One that I love personally:** Tara Brach, *Radical Compassion: Learning to Love Yourself and Your World with the Practice of RAIN* (New York: Penguin Life, 2019).

CHAPTER 10: FINDING THE ANSR AND LETTING YOUR BODY BE YOUR PROOF

177 **"The Guest House":** Rumi, "The Guest House."
178 **"little shmoos":** Ram Dass, *Be Here Now* (New York: Harmony Books, 1978).

CHAPTER 12: SELF-COMPASSION AND ACCEPTANCE AS ESSENTIAL TOOLS

212 **Dr. Kristin Neff:** Kristin Neff, PhD, *Self-Compassion: The Proven Power of Being Kind to Yourself* (New York: Morrow, 2015).
216 **Buddhism teaches:** Thich Nhat Hanh. *The Heart of the Buddha's Teaching: Transforming Suffering into Peace, Joy, and Liberation* (New York: Harmony Books, 1999).
218 **"Autobiography in Five Short Chapters":** Portia Nelson, "An Autobiography in Five Short Chapters," *There's a Hole in My Sidewalk: The Romance of Self-Discovery* (New York: Atria Books, 1977).
219 **Now that you know better:** Janet Lowe, *Oprah Winfrey Speaks: Insights from the World's Most Influential Voice* (New York: Wiley, 1998).
220 **I often reference:** Danielle LaPorte, *White Hot Truth: Clarity for Keeping It Real on Your Spiritual Path—from One Seeker to Another* (Vancouver, Canada: Virtuonica, 2017).
221 **As spiritual innovator Byron Katie:** "Byron Katie > Quotes > Quotable Quote," Goodreads, accessed March 7, 2024, https://www

.goodreads.com/quotes/132449-when-you-argue-with-reality-you -lose-but-only-100.

CHAPTER 14: TAKE BACK YOUR POWER

247 **As the brilliant philosopher:** Joseph Campbell, *The Hero with a Thousand Faces* (New York: Pantheon Books, 1949).

254 **What if, as the mystic poet Rumi wrote:** "Rumi (Jalal ad-Din Muhammad ar-Rumi) > Quotes > Quotable Quote," Goodreads, accessed March 9, 2024, https://www.goodreads.com/quotes/1299504 -i-said-what-about-my-eyes-he-said-keep-them.

INDEX